JUST THE FACTS

~

ABORTION A-Z

Michele C. Moore and Caroline M. de Costa

Order this book online at www.trafford.com/06-3146
or email orders@trafford.com

Most Trafford titles are also available at major online book retailers.

Note for Librarians: A cataloguing record for this book is available from Library
and Archives Canada at www.collectionscanada.ca/amicus/index-e.html

ISBN: 978-1-4251-1387-2

*We at Trafford believe that it is the responsibility of us all, as both individuals
and corporations, to make choices that are environmentally and socially sound.
You, in turn, are supporting this responsible conduct each time you purchase a
Trafford book, or make use of our publishing services. To find out how you are
helping, please visit www.trafford.com/responsiblepublishing.html*

*Our mission is to efficiently provide the world's finest, most comprehensive
book publishing service, enabling every author to experience success.
To find out how to publish your book, your way, and have it available
worldwide, visit us online at www.trafford.com/10510*

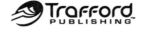

www.trafford.com

North America & international
toll-free: 1 888 232 4444 (USA & Canada)
phone: 250 383 6864 ♦ fax: 250 383 6804
email: info@trafford.com

The United Kingdom & Europe
phone: +44 (0)1865 722 113 ♦ local rate: 0845 230 9601
facsimile: +44 (0)1865 722 868 ♦ email: info.uk@trafford.com

10 9 8 7 6 5 4

Disclaimer: although the authors have made every effort to be comprehensive in their search for facts about abortion, it is inevitable that some facts may have been overlooked or have been unavailable to the authors at the time of writing. If you find such a lack, please contact the authors so that it may be remedied in future editions of this book.

We thank the many women we have cared for who have allowed us to share their stories in this book. Also our families, who have been so supportive of all our writing together. We would also like to thank Cait Calcutt of 'Children by Choice' in Brisbane, Australia for her assistance with the preparation of this book.

Introduction

Every year, millions of women conceive unplanned and unwanted pregnancies, and have to consider for themselves whether or not they are able to, or wish to, continue the pregnancy. Whether women have any options in this matter depends greatly on where they live: this may be in countries where safe abortion is easily accessible and financially realistic, but for large numbers of women this is not the case. Safe abortion is available by law to women in the United States and Canada, as it is in most of Europe, the United Kingdom, China, Australia and many other countries. It is available with variable legal rulings in a number of others, but in many abortion remains illegal except to save the woman's life, and in some places not even in that situation. Women in European countries such as Ireland, Malta and Poland, for example, need to travel outside national borders to access safe abortion. Even in countries where abortion is legal, its physical accessibility varies greatly between regions and between urban and rural areas. Examples include the US, Canada and Australia, where several states or provinces have very limited numbers of abortion providers, and women need to know of the existence of services, and be able to travel long distances, if they are to access safe legal abortion.

Currently threatening the accessibility of safe abortion in several countries is the abortion 'debate' – really not a debate at all, but the diametrically opposed views of pro-choice versus pro-life advocates. As any television viewer settling down to watch such a 'debate' well knows, there is little possibility of compromise between these groups because they are philosophically at opposite poles. The only common thread is the wish of both groups for a reduction in the number of induced abortions performed. However, their approaches to this goal differ enormously, with the pro-choice group advocating better access to reliable birth control methods, and more education about these, and many of the pro-life groups advocating sexual abstinence. Whether conciliation can come about in the shared purpose of preventing unwanted pregnancies remains to be seen.

Until the beginning of the nineteenth century, abortion, although forbidden completely by some religions and in some circumstances by others, was not a crime. Criminalization of abortion came about in the US, Britain and other countries in the course of the nineteenth century, ostensibly in the interests of women's health. Abortion remained on the criminal statute books in these countries for more than one hundred years, until the movements for reform and repeal of abortion laws of the second half of the twentieth century succeeded in bringing about safe legal abortion, accessible in principle to all women.

The history of abortion over the past century and a half, from so-called 'back alleys' to parliaments in Britain and Continental Europe, and to the United States Supreme Court, is the history of many women's personal tragedies and suffering. Men are not the main protagonists in this story, although they had a major role in restricting access to safe, legal abortion for women for many years, in criminalizing procedures and enforcing abortion laws. However many men also played a role in the sympathetic provision of abortions for women, during the century in which the procedure was illegal, and supported efforts to bring about law repeal and reform, in the United States, Canada, the United Kingdom, Australia and elsewhere.

Currently in the United States, there are frequent attempts to limit the existing rights of women to access safe abortion. The past five years have seen the restriction of Medicaid coverage of mifepristone, effectively limiting access to this drug for low-income women, and restrictions to some forms of late abortion in several US states. Conservative appointments to the Supreme Court raise the possibility of the Roe vs. Wade decision, which in 1973 granted access to safe abortion to American women, being overturned. Women's access to abortion services in the US should not be taken for granted even though a majority of the population believes that abortion is a matter for a woman and her doctor and do not favor encompassing bans such as some of those proposed for late abortion. In Canada women do not yet have access to mifepristone. In Italy, efforts continue to bring about access of Italian women to medical abortion; elsewhere in Europe, in Malta, Poland and Portugal, women's access to all forms of abortion is extremely limited. In Australia also, efforts continue to bring about the introduction of mifepristone-previous legislation banning the use and import of the drug has been lifted, although it is not yet widely available. There are also ongoing attempts in Australia to remove state laws on abortion from the criminal codes, where they remain despite the fact that around 80% of the Australian population believe that women should be able to access safe abortion. These continuing threats to hard-won rights, and the illegality of abortion in many of the less-advantaged countries of the world, mean that it is important women everywhere stay well-informed about developments in abortion politics.

We wish to address these topics in a balanced and non-judgmental way. We also believe that women need knowledge of methods of abortion and of which particular methods are appropriate at different stages of pregnancy. They need to know how to obtain information about counseling and abortion services in their own particular geographic area and what laws and restrictions exist in that area. They need to know the risks and complications of the different methods of abortion and how having an abortion may affect their subsequent health. They need to know what research has been done on long-term sequelae of various methods, and what services are available to them in aftercare.

There are many books available on abortion. Some are excellent and we provide a list of these in our bibliography. Many are unashamedly political arguments for one side or another in the 'debate.' This is perfectly all right provided the authors make their bias clear to the reader, however unfortunately many of them distort medical facts and figures to support their own viewpoints. As well, we have found that most unbiased books on the topic directed at non-medical readers deal only with certain aspects of abortion, usually history, while not providing much medical information.

There is also an abundance of information on the Internet. However medical information on the Internet is not subject to the same kind of peer-review as books published by reputable publishers nor does it usually provide thoughtful interpretation of complex medical facts and data.

Abortion continues to be a subject widely discussed and is likely to continue to be the subject of political maneuvring in the foreseeable future particularly in the US and

Australia. While this discussion continues, methods of medical termination of pregnancy continue to improve, as do methods of contraception, and in this climate, women will continue to need concise, accurate and non-judgmental information. It is for these reasons that we have decided to write this book and to format it as an A – Z. This will enable anyone to access the information that she is looking for, in a limited or a comprehensive manner.

Yes, we are broadly pro-choice. As medical students in Dublin, Ireland in the 1960s and 70s, we saw firsthand the sad results when women do not have access to safe abortion: death, chronic ill-health, enforced pregnancy and 'shotgun' marriages. We have described some of these in our book. As doctors, we have cared for women in one way and another, in obstetrics and gynecology and women's health, ever since we began practice – our combined experience covers more than sixty years. We believe firmly that a woman has a right to as much accurate information as possible about her body, and about what her health choices might be. We also believe that if a woman chooses to terminate her pregnancy then that decision should be made by herself in conjunction with her doctor. We hope to provide information that will help a woman in choosing for herself. In addition the book provides a great deal of information about the history of the abortion movement worldwide and the politics involved.

For every abortion statistic there is a woman. And so interwoven with the alphabetical information are the stories of some women we have cared for. Names and other details have been changed to protect identities but the stories are real and we thank all these women for sharing their experiences with us. We have included these stories to show that all kinds of women, of all ages, single, married, divorced, widowed, in many different occupations and lifestyle situations, practicing a particular religion, or not, can find themselves having to make a choice about abortion for themselves. An A-Z of women, you could say, and that is what you will find, from Alanna through to Zoe. Through these stories, we show the human aspect of the experience of abortion and the difficulties involved in making a decision for or against the procedure. While most of the stories involve a decision for abortion, some are about women who chose to continue with their pregnancies, either to keep and rear their child, or to have the child adopted.

In our appendices you will find a list of resources in the United States, the United Kingdom, Australia and elsewhere, and some suggestions for further reading. Our aim is to provide a comprehensive guide to the subject for non-medical readers – while the book is mostly addressed to women we hope it may also be useful to those men who choose to consult it. While we see our readership as living mostly in North America, we believe the information we have provided about abortion itself, and the stories, are universally applicable. We have also endeavored to provide some information about the legal status of abortion and abortion resources in other countries. We would be very receptive to suggestions about material to include in future editions of this book.

Chronology

1803 – English Omnibus Crime Act made abortion illegal at any stage of pregnancy

1821 – first American state law on abortion, designed to protect mothers

1857 – Texas makes abortion or attempted abortion illegal

1861 – the British Offences Against the Person Act was passed in Britain ostensibly to protect women from unsafe abortion practices. This Act became the basis of law in Australian colonies and other parts of the British Empire and was subsequently incorporated into criminal laws in many of these places

1873 – anti-obscenity laws in US Congress outlaw importation of, advertisement of, and use of the mails to send contraceptive devices. Not repealed until mid-1900s

1916 – First birth control clinic opened by Margaret Sanger in NYC

1921 – American Birth Control League founded by Margaret Sanger

1936 – ALRA –Abortion Law Reform Association formed in England

1937 – American Medical Association comes out in favor of birth control.

1942 – American Birth Control League becomes the Planned Parenthood Federation of America.

1950 – 1970 abortion law reform movement in US, UK and elsewhere

1960 – AMA reports abortion ban unenforceable

1962 – AMA approves therapeutic abortion provisions. Thalidomide pregnancy case. (Sherry Finkbein)

1965 – Griswold v. Connecticut rubella epidemic leads to increased demand for therapeutic abortion. Planned Parenthood sues CT and wins against anti-contraception laws.

1967 – California, Colorado and North Carolina enact reformed abortion laws. United Kingdom – introduction of Abortion Act, legalized abortion in England, Scotland and Wales

1969 – National Abortion Rights Action League founded
 Menhennit Ruling – a legal ruling in Melbourne, Australia which allowed doctors to perform abortions in certain circumstances

1970 – Roe v. Wade filed, also Doe – cases consolidated

1971 – Dr. Jane Hodgson convicted for performing in-hospital abortion.

1972 – Eisenstadt v. Baird – US Supreme Court held that constitutional right to privacy applies equally to unmarried people as to married, making it unconstitutional to deny contraceptive information, articles, or drugs to unmarried people.

1973 – Supreme Court decision in Roe v. Wade – right to abortion is found in the Due Process Clause; the state has interest in life of fetus after first trimester but must pass the 'strict scrutiny' standard. Justice Harry Blackmun announced majority view, Justices Rehnquist and White dissented

1973 – Doe v. Bolton – US Supreme Court found Georgia law unconstitutional because it unduly restricted woman's right to choose.

1973 – American Right to Life Committee founded

1975 – Bigelow v. Virginia – advertisement of abortion services is found to be protected under the First Amendment.

1976 – Planned Parenthood of Central Missouri v. Danforth – Supreme Court allows written informed consent requirements by states but strikes down Missouri requirements for spousal and parental consent.

Justice John Paul Stevens joins court – supports Roe.

1977 – Hyde Amendment passed into law – denies federal funds for abortion

1977 – Carey v. Population Services – held unconstitutional a New York law criminalizing dispensing contraceptives to minors under 16, advertising or displaying contraceptives and requiring that only pharmacists dispense contraceptives.

1977 – Beal v. Doe and Maher v. Roe – US Supreme Court upheld the policies of Pennsylvania and Connecticut that limit the use of public funds to only those abortions deemed 'medically necessary.'

1977 – Poelker v. Doe – as above but re Missouri.

1980 – Ronald Reagan wins presidential election, calling for an anti-abortion amendment to the Constitution. Supreme Court upholds ban on federal funding for abortion. In challenge before the Supreme Court, Hyde Amendment is upheld.

1981 – Justice Sandra Day-O'Connor joins Supreme Court and will be swing vote on abortion issues.

1982 – First abortion clinic bombing

1983 – City of Akron v. Akron Center for Reproductive Health – Supreme Court invalidated Akron requirements that D&E abortions be performed only in hospitals, that informed consent materials include the clause 'an unborn child is a human life from the moment of conception', parental consent requirements without an adequate waiver provision, 24-hour waiting period requirements, and requirements regarding disposal of the fetal remains.

1983 – Planned Parenthood Association of Kansas City v. Ashcroft – the Court upheld Kansas requirements that two doctors be present during later term abortions, that parental consent or judicial waiver be required for minor women, and that pathology reports be filed after abortions. It struck down the provision that all second-trimester abortions be performed in hospitals.

1983 – Simopoulis v. Virginia – Supreme Court upheld the conviction of a doctor who performed a second-trimester abortion outside of a licensed hospital, noting that the definition of 'hospital' differed between the Missouri and Virginia law.

1986 – Justice Antonin Scalia joins the Supreme Court and will be Roe's most adamant critic.

1986 – Thornburgh v. American College of Obstetricians and Gynecologists – a direct challenge to Roe v. Wade. The Court struck down provisions requiring doctors to give women antiabortion information, permitting disclosure of doctor/patient information and post-viability 'degree of care' obligations to preserve the life of the 'unborn child.'

1987 – First 'rescue' by Randall Terry

1988 – Operation Rescue founded

1988 – Justice Anthony Kennedy joins the Supreme Court. Clinics receiving Title X federal funding enjoined from discussing abortion with clients.

1989 – Majority opinion of the Supreme Court drops the 'fundamental right' language of Roe. Requires that state laws be rational. Upholds Missouri restrictions on abortions (Webster v. Reproductive Health Services). Justice O'Connor stands up for Roe.

1990 – Hodgson v. Minnesota – Court held that the requirement for two parent notification is unconstitutional without a judicial waiver provision. In Ohio v. Akron Center for Reproductive Health the parental consent provision was upheld because provision was made for an alternate judicial waiver.

1991 – Justice David Souter joins the Court. Court upholds instructions limiting speech in clinics receiving Title X funds (Rust v. Sullivan). Justice O'Connor dissents.

1992 – Justice Clarence Thomas added to Court. PA rules on abortion upheld by the Court. Attempt to reverse Roe defeated by Justices Kennedy, O'Connor, Souter, Stevens and Blackmun.

Planned Parenthood of Southeastern Pennsylvania v. Casey – Court upheld provisions requiring doctors to provide information on adoption and on health risks related to abortion. It also upheld 24-hour waiting periods and single parent consent requirements for minor women.

1992 – Bill Clinton wins Presidency as a pro-choice candidate.

1993 – Clinton lifts the gag rule in Title X programs. Justice Ruth Bader Ginsburg joins the Court. Congress votes to allow federal funding of abortions in cases of reported rape or incest.

Escalation of abortion clinic violence in the murder of Dr. David Gunn

Bray v. Alexandria Women's Health Clinic – Court finds that antiabortion activists were not engaged in gender-based discrimination.

1994 – Freedom of Access to Clinic Entrances Act passed.

Justice Stephen Breyer joins the Supreme Court.

Court finds that buffer zone around clinic entrances is not a violation of free speech. Court finds that federal anti-racketeering laws can be used against antiabortion conspiracies.

Dr. John Britton and Lt.Col. (Ret.) James Barrett are murdered by Paul Hill.

Shannon Lowry and Leann Nichols are murdered by John Salvi, III.

Freedom of Access to Clinic Entrances Law – a law passed by Congress, making it a crime to block access to abortion clinics and mandating penalties for harming anyone during demonstrations at clinics.

1997 – Mazurek v. Armstrong – held that state requirements that all abortions be performed by physicians are constitutional.

1998 – Dr. Barnett Slepian murdered by James Kopp; Officer Robert Sanderson murdered by Eric Rudolph.

2001 – Unborn Victims Act becomes law – makes it a federal crime to harm a fetus in an assault on a pregnant woman.

Bush administration restricts Medicaid coverage of RU-486 to those cases involving rape or incest or endangerment to the life of the mother.

Pres. Bush issues an executive order directing AID to halt federal funding for family planning groups that support abortion overseas.

2003 – Partial Birth Abortion Act passed into law. The language of the Act allows for no exception for medical necessity and states that this type of abortion is never medically necessary. Challenge will be heard by the Supreme Court in 2006/2007.

2005 – Death of Chief Justice Rehnquist, John Roberts appointed Chief Justice. Roberts' record indicates he is pro-life.

2006 – Sandra Day O'Connor retired and Samuel Alito, known to be pro-life, was appointed as her successor

2007 - US Supreme Court found that the Partial Birth Abortion Act is constitutional.

The A-Z follows. **Bold type** is used to indicate that a topic referred to in an entry has a separate entry.

A

Alanna

Life couldn't have been better. Darren and I were happily married and as much in love as when we were teenagers and our two children were healthy and seemed to be nice little individuals. We planned to have one more before we turned thirty-five and figured that this would be the year. We had bought a home three years before and were able to swing all the expenses because we both had very good jobs. Anyway, our planning worked because I had just found out that I was pregnant.

When Darren heard our good news, he said we must take a weekend holiday before we were back in diapers again. My mother was happy to come and stay with the kids and so it was planned.

Mom had arrived at the house to prepare supper for the kids that Friday night so that Darren and I could take off as soon as he returned from work. In fact, she opened the door to a State Trooper. He told me there had been an accident and Darren had been taken to the hospital; he had come to take me there.

I'll never forget that room where I waited or the smell. The room had no windows and the walls were green. There was a heavy smell of antiseptics and the whole place was stifling. I noted the number of holes in the ceiling tiles and tried to think of everything but why the doctors were taking so long. Eventually, a doctor entered the room: Emerson Brown, MD, his pocket patch said. He said he was very sorry, he and the staff had done all that they could but Darren – my Darren – was just too grievously injured and had not responded to the resuscitation efforts. I was numb and I couldn't understand what this very kind man was trying to tell me.

Somehow, I got home and my mother took over. She helped make funeral arrangements, handled well-meaning friends and relatives and got us through the next few weeks. Finally the day came when I awoke to realize that I was now a pregnant young widow with two little children, a mortgage and a job that had helped support our lifestyle but that wouldn't keep us afloat now. There was very little health insurance; we were young and healthy and could foresee no need. Mom certainly was willing to help but her health wasn't good enough for me to hand over much of my burden to her.

I went to talk with the financial adviser at the bank and we drew up a budget. I earn just enough to make all our payments and keep the kids and me fed and clothed. There is no extra for vacations or frills and if a major appliance breaks down, I'll have to draw on the small amount of insurance we received. I've invested it so that there will be at least a little something for the kids' education. There was no possibility that I could swing this and be pregnant. Realizing this just floored me and I was again ill with grief.

I'm so lucky in my mother; she arranged for our pastor, Rev. Egan, to come and counsel me. Rev. Egan is warm and strong and listened to me with an open heart and sometimes encompassing arms and helped me come to the terrible decision to abort this pregnancy.

My abortion was not physically difficult; I was nine weeks pregnant at the time. It was, however, a terrible blow to deliberately lose the child that Darren and I had conceived in love, but I know today that the children and I could not have made it in those very difficult years after Darren's death if I had had another child. As it was, there were times we had to visit the local food shelf to stretch my pay check a little further.

A

Aberration – an abnormality or imperfection. Often used to refer to **chromosomal** aberration or anomaly, for example, Down syndrome or trisomy 21, which may be a medical reason for an abortion.

Abortifacient – a drug, or a chemical or herbal compound, that induces abortion. **RU-486 (mifepristone)** is an example of such a drug.

Abortion – the expulsion or removal of the contents of the pregnant uterus (womb) prior to the time when the **embryo** or **fetus** is able to live without the assistance of the mother's body. (An embryo means a developing baby from the time of conception up to eight weeks of pregnancy; a fetus refers to the developing baby from eight weeks of pregnancy until birth.) An abortion may be a spontaneous natural event, when it is often referred to as a miscarriage – physicians may call it a 'spontaneous abortion.' It may also be brought about by the intervention of another person, by surgical or medical means, with the intention of ending the pregnancy – an induced abortion. The **Centers for Disease Control** define a legal abortion as 'a procedure, performed by a licensed physician or someone acting under the supervision of a licensed physician, that was intended to terminate a suspected or known intrauterine pregnancy and to produce a nonviable fetus at any gestational age.'

> **accidental abortion** – abortion caused by injury e.g. road crash, domestic violence

> **aspiration abortion** – induced abortion performed by using a narrow plastic tube (cannula) passed into the uterus via the canal of the cervix, and using suction to remove the uterine contents, either with a hand operated pump (manual aspiration) or an electrical suction pump

> **atraumatic abortion** – usually refers to abortion by **menstrual aspiration**.

> **complete abortion** – expulsion of the fetus, placenta and membranes

> **elective abortion** – an induced abortion performed at the request of the mother, in the absence of a medical reason for the abortion. This is also called voluntary abortion or abortion on demand.

> **habitual abortion** – this does not refer to induced abortion, but rather to repetitive (more than three) spontaneous abortions or miscarriages.

> **incomplete abortion** – some of the 'products of conception' – e.g. part of the fetus, membranes or placenta, are left inside the uterus. This can be a cause of bleeding and infection. This is more common with spontaneous abortions than with induced abortions and with illegal abortions performed by untrained persons.

> **infected abortion** – abortion accompanied or followed by fever, pelvic pain and abnormal vaginal discharge and with an elevation of the white blood cell count. This is not uncommon in illegal abortions.

> **medical abortion** – process of expulsion of the products of conception using drugs (**mifepristone, methotrexate, misoprostol, gemeprost**)

> **partial-birth abortion** – this is a popular, non-medical term for a late termination of pregnancy. Labor is induced by conventional methods (see **induction of labor**) but

before 24 and usually before 20 weeks of pregnancy. If the head of the fetus is born first – a cephalic presentation – delivery proceeds as it would in a normal delivery. If the fetus is in a breech presentation, once the fetus is delivered as far as the chest or neck the contents of the skull of the fetus may be evacuated by a suction catheter and the skull decompressed, allowing for an easier vaginal delivery. The fetus is born before the time at which it can live independently from the mother. The term may also be applied to the medical procedure used for late abortions known as **Dilation and extraction** or **D&X**. The term is used in legislation outlawing some late terminations, which was passed by Congress on 21 October 2003, and by many states before and since that date; this legislation has since been limited or blocked in many states. See also **Partial-Birth Abortion Laws** and **Partial –Birth Abortion Laws, statements of professional bodies on.**

 saline-induced abortion – an abortion induced by injecting a strong (20 – 25%) saline solution into the sac around the fetus. This was usually done in a second **trimester** abortion to induce labor, but has fallen into disfavor because of occasional serious complications, including DIC (disseminated intravascular coagulation) and maternal death.

 septic abortion – an infected abortion accompanied by a generalized blood-borne infection. This is life-threatening and is more common after illegal abortions done under less than ideal conditions.

 surgical abortion – procedure carried out using a suction cannula or instruments to remove the fetus, placenta and membranes from the uterine cavity, followed by curettage of the inside walls of the uterus to remove any remaining tissue. See also **vacuum aspiration.**

 therapeutic abortion – abortion done before the fetus is viable in order to safeguard the physical or mental health of the mother. This is also called justifiable or eugenic abortion.

Abortion Act, United Kingdom, 1967. Legalized abortion in England, Wales and Scotland, does not apply in Northern Ireland. With some modifications is the law under which abortions are now performed in the United Kingdom. Induced abortion can be performed in situations where continuing the pregnancy poses a greater risk to the life or physical or mental health of the woman, or her existing family or children, than if abortion is carried out. It can also be performed when the fetus is shown to have a serious abnormality. Two medical practitioners must agree that the abortion is indicated, abortion can only be performed by a registered medical practitioner (although drugs to induce a medical abortion can be given by a registered nurse under the direction of a physician), the certificates signed by the two medical practitioners must be kept for three years and all abortions must be notified to the UK Department of Health so that accurate statistics are available. . Abortion both surgical and medical is widely available throughout the United Kingdom with the exception of Northern Ireland, both in **NHS** hospitals and through private organizations such as **BPAS.**

Abortion Law Reform Association – ALRA. Formed in England in 1936, by women who were mostly middle-class, with leftist/feminist leanings, ALRA was also supported by working class women in its demands for legal, safe abortion. ALRA was integral to the campaign that led to the 1967 Abortion Act in the United Kingdom; the association's aim was to legalize unsafe illegal abortions that were already occurring. Abortion-by-choice was not part of their program.

Abortion Rights Coalition of Canada – pro-choice organization active in lobbying for increased abortion rights awareness.

Abortionist – one who performs abortions, usually refers to illegal abortions.

Abortion Mortality Surveillance System – this part of the CDC attempts to identify all abortion-related deaths. It defines an abortion-related death as a death resulting from 1) a direct complication of an abortion, 2) an indirect complication caused by the chain of events initiated by the abortion or 3) an aggravation of a pre-existing condition by the physiologic or psychological effects of the abortion, regardless of the amount of time between the abortion and the death.

Abortion provider – the term currently used to describe a person, normally a qualified medical practitioner, performing an induced abortion.

Abortus – a technical term referring to the fetus or embryo expelled in early pregnancy, with all of its accompanying tissues. By definition the fetus weighs less than 500 gm and measures less than 25 cm from the heel to the crown of the head.

Abstinence – refraining voluntarily from sexual activity. This is the method of birth control advocated by many conservative Christians.

ACOG – see **American College of Obstetrician and Gynecologists**

ACT – see **Australian Capital Territory**

Activists – persons who are actively involved in efforts to influence the legal availability of abortion, utilizing the media, politics and advocacy to further their cause. There are activists on both sides of the abortion question. Individuals will be cited separately with their particular noteworthy actions.

Age, of consent – legal definition of the age at which an individual is deemed capable of making a marriage contract or of engaging willingly in sexual activity. Depending on the country and/or state, this is usually between 14 and 18 years of age. It is much younger in some countries. See also **consenting adolescent**.

gestational age – the age of a fetus or embryo in weeks, starting from the first day of the mother's last period.

Alabama – rated F by **NARAL**. Pre- Roe ban on abortion still in force, last amended in 1975. AL code 13A - 13-7. AL code 26-23-1 to 26-23-6 (1997) outlaws abortions performed after twelve weeks unless necessary to preserve the mother's life. No language in the law provides for the health of the mother. 7% of AL counties have an abortion provider. State law mandates counseling by a physician or other specified professional, such counseling to include 1) the nature of the procedure, including risks and alternatives, 2) the gestational age of the fetus and its 3) anatomical and physiological characteristics at that gestational age, 4) that if the fetus is of a viable age, the mother has the right to request an abortion method likely to preserve the life of the unborn baby and to use all reasonable methods to preserve the life of the child, 5) the physician must perform an ultrasound prior to abortion and the woman has the right to see this ultrasound, 6) she has the right to view a state-prepared video, 7) she is free to withdraw consent at any time without loss of state or federally-funded benefits, and 8) the name of the physician who will perform the abortion is to be provided in writing. Also, the woman must be provided with state-prepared materials by a designated professional at least 24 hours prior to the abortion. These materials reiterate the risks of abortion and provide alternative resources to help the woman who should decide to keep her child or offer the child for adoption.

Public funding for abortion is limited to those women whose lives are endangered by continuing the pregnancy or those pregnancies resulting from rape or incest. Emergency contraception is available in state department of public health clinics.

Alan Guttmacher Institute – a non-profit group specializing in reproductive research, policy analysis and public education. The stated mission of the Institute is 'to protect the reproductive choices of all women and men in the United States and throughout the world, supporting their ability to obtain the information and services needed to achieve their full human rights, safeguard their health and exercise their individual responsibilities in regard to sexual behavior and relationships, reproduction and family formation.' The Institute was founded in 1968 by Alan Guttmacher, MD, (1898 – 1974), who had formerly been president of the Planned Parenthood Foundation of America. The data generated by the Institute is accepted as accurate by both pro-choice and pro-life advocates.

Alaska – rated A by **NARAL**. The Alaska Constitution protects the right to reproductive choice as a fundamental right. Alaska enacted a ban on abortions after 12 weeks, Alaska statute 18.16.050 (1997) but this ban has been declared unconstitutional under the state constitution. Under a law passed in 2004, a woman may not have an abortion until a designated health professional has 1) informed the woman of the name of the physician who will perform the procedure and the gestational age of her fetus and 2) provided the required state-prepared written materials or described the proposed procedure and the risks attendant upon it. These requirements may be bypassed only in cases of medical emergency, rape or incest. Alaskan law requires consent of one parent before any woman under age 17 who is not emancipated may have an abortion. Public funds may be used for medically necessary abortions. Pharmacists are allowed to provide emergency contraception directly to women without a prescription.

AMA – see **American Medical Association**

Amenorrhoea – absence of menstruation.

 primary amenorrhoea – failure to begin to menstruate by age 16 (some authorities say age 18)

 secondary amenorrhoea – stopping of periods for at least 3 months in a woman of reproductive age who has previously had periods. Pregnancy is the most common cause.

American College of Obstetricians and Gynecologists (ACOG) – the national professional organization of specialists, with 40,000 members. ACOG is committed to promoting and maintaining the highest standards of ethical practice in women's health. ACOG has issued numerous statements and guidelines for the practice of abortion including *Medical Management of Abortion*, a detailed evidence-based resource to guide practitioners in decision making and the performance of abortions. ACOG has also taken a political role in regard to abortion including statements on **Partial-Birth Abortion Laws** and on low maternal mortality rates in association with legal abortion.

American Medical Association – a professional association of physicians and surgeons in the United States to promote mutual interests and concerns. In the nineteenth and early twentieth century, this influential organization actively opposed abortion, primarily because of concern for the safety of women exposed to the procedure as then practiced. The official position of the AMA today is that it is ethical for doctors to perform abortion in accordance with state and federal laws. The AMA supported the passage of the 'Partial

Birth Abortion Ban Act of 1997' as long as provision was made to safeguard the life of the mother, that the banned procedure was clearly defined, and that any physician accused under the Ban have the right to have his/her conduct reviewed by a State Medical Board prior to any criminal proceedings. The AMA has opposed requirements that doctors counsel patients with state-dictated materials on the basis that it interferes with doctor-patient interaction.

Amniocentesis – a diagnostic procedure in which a needle is introduced through the abdominal wall into the sac around the developing fetus and a small amount of amniotic fluid is drawn off to be tested for chromosomal abnormalities. This is usually done around the 16th week of pregnancy. If abnormalities are detected, the mother may opt for a therapeutic abortion.

Analgesia – pain relief. Abortions, both surgical and medical, are accompanied by pain to some degree. Surgical abortion is usually performed, in countries where it is legal, using either local or general anesthesia. Medical abortion should include the provision of adequate pain relief including drugs such as pethidine (meperidine), codeine, paracetamol and non-steroidal inflammatories such as naproxen. Medical abortion during the second trimester may be particularly painful and epidural analgesia is often appropriate.

Anesthesia – the absence of pain. Anesthesia either local or general is desirable for the safe performance of surgical abortion. For surgical abortion under local anesthetic, a drug such as lidocaine is injected into the cervix and around the nerves supplying the cervix '(paracervical block'), thereby numbing the area. Treatment with a drug such as naproxen (or other **Non Steroidal Anti Inflammatory Drug**) two hours prior to the abortion procedure may increase the effects of local anesthesia. Self-administered nitrous oxide gas, which provides pain relief without permitting the woman to lose consciousness, has also been used in some centers in conjunction with local anesthesia. General anesthesia is produced by a number of different drugs and must be administered by a specialist anesthetist or other physician with appropriate training; in some countries general anesthesia is administered by nurse-practitioners under the supervision of a physician. General anesthesia requires that the woman be fasting prior to surgery and remain under medical/nursing observation for some hours post-op.

Antibiotics – drugs used to prevent or treat infections caused by bacteria. Antibiotics are frequently given at the time of performing a surgical abortion, to treat certain sexually transmitted infections (specifically Chlamydia and/or gonorrhea) and to prevent infection of the uterine cavity, fallopian tubes and surrounding tissues following the abortion process. They may also be given to treat infection occurring post-abortion including infection that has spread outside the pelvis (see septic abortion). The antibiotics most commonly used in association with abortion are penicillins, metronidazole and doxycycline. Antibiotics are also being used increasingly in conjunction with medical abortion to prevent infection although there is no specific medical evidence to support this procedure.

Arizona – rated C+ by **NARAL**. The pre-Roe ban on abortion has never been repealed, so technically abortion is illegal and subject to penalty in AZ, although this ban has been found unconstitutional and unenforceable. Certain organizations receiving state funds are prohibited from counseling or referring women for abortion services. The Arizona Board of Regents prohibits abortion in any university facility unless it is necessary to preserve the mother's life. Any woman under the age of 18 must have the written consent of one parent unless she certifies that the pregnancy is the result of sexual abuse by a near family member, knowing that this will be reported to law. Arizona requires any insurance plan that covers prescription drugs to provide equitable coverage for contraception. It allows state funds to be used for abortion for eligible women if the abortion is medically necessary. The State Constitution of Arizona protects reproductive rights.

Arkansas – rated F by **NARAL**, has not repealed its pre-Roe ban on abortion. This was held unconstitutional as applied to abortion performed by physicians. Mandatory counseling and delay are very similar to those in **Alabama**. State employee insurance plans will not cover abortion unless it is necessary to preserve the mother's life. State law requires notarized written consent of a parent for any woman under 18 who is not emancipated to have an abortion. Any use of public funds for abortion is prohibited except when the mother's life is endangered or the pregnancy is the result of rape or incest. Arkansas State Constitution amendment 68 (1988) states that 'the policy of Arkansas is to protect the life of every unborn child conception until birth, to the extent permitted by the Federal Constitution.'

Army of God – militant anti-abortion group. Members have been involved in violence against abortion providers and clinics and have advocated violence as justified to "prevent the deaths of unborn babies."

Ascherman's syndrome – a rare condition that may follow curettage of the uterus for induced abortion or removal of tissue remaining from a spontaneous abortion. Normally curettage removes only the surface lining of the uterus; if the deeper layers are removed the tissue cannot regenerate in future menstrual cycles, preventing the possibility of future pregnancy. Scar tissue grows across the cavity of the uterus and periods usually stop or become very scanty. Treatment consists of cutting away the scar tissue and keeping the cavity of the uterus open with an intra-uterine device for some months, however this is not always successful.

Aspiration – removal of material by suction.

   menstrual aspiration – suction of the lining of the uterus performed 1 to 3 weeks after a missed period, with or without a positive pregnancy test. Also called atraumatic abortion, menstrual extraction, menstrual induction and mini-abortion.

   vacuum aspiration – term used to describe surgical abortion using a cannula attached to a vacuum suction apparatus.

Aspirator – any device used to remove material from a body cavity by suction.

Australian Capital Territory – The Health Regulation (Maternal Health Information) Act 1998 (ACT), which was designed to clarify requirements for abortion and to decriminalize the procedure, specifies that abortions must only be performed by appropriately qualified persons 'in suitable premises.' The woman must be provided with specified advice, information and referral about abortion and the woman and the doctor must sign a declaration that she has received this. There is a 72 hour 'cooling-off' period during which a woman can change her mind about her decision for abortion. Abortion is provided in a free-standing clinic.

Australian Medical Association, position on abortion – 2006 revision of 1998 Reproductive Health and Reproductive Technology position statement respects the rights of doctors to hold differing views regarding the termination of pregnancy; recommends that where the law permits induced abortion this should be performed by appropriately trained medical practitioners in approved premises; supports the introduction of medical abortion and advises that doctors should counsel women requesting such information about the risks both of continuing the pregnancy and of undergoing abortion.

Avery, Byllye – founder of National Black Women's Health Project in 1983 in response to issues affecting the health of black women.

B

Betty

Oh, it is just such a common and sordid little story and I'm ashamed of myself for being so naive, but there you have it.

I was in my first year at college. I felt very liberated and free of the constraints of my upbringing by my well-meaning, but bitterly poor and pious cousin and his wife. They were very good to take me in when my folks were killed when I was ten, but it was a hard situation for all of us. Winning a full scholarship to college was like winning the lottery for me.

Part of my financial aid was a college work/study job and I took a position with one of the professors. He was my French professor and I thought he was very kind. All he required was some photocopying and filing, not much else. At least at first. By November, he had begun stroking my hand and nibbling at my ear, and by December, he had seduced me. It probably wasn't hard because I was so very green. He invited me out to a dark little restaurant for an intimate dinner, complete with wine, and then took me back to his office. I liked the kissing but when he pushed me back on the sofa, right on top of piles of papers and pulled my clothes off, I became alarmed and begged him to stop. He didn't and after he said that he knew I was just acting out in order to further excite him. He said I was a hot little piece. It never occurred to me that he might have a wife tucked away or that anything other than true love forever was on the menu.

In February, I missed my period and when I started throwing up after each meal, I caught on. Not even I was so stupid that I could ignore these signs. Somehow, I didn't think it would happen, though; I thought he was protecting me.

When I told him my suspicions, he was infuriated and accused me of trying to trap him. Didn't I know he had a family, he asked?

I was devastated. How could I have done this thing? Did I chase him? Was it all my fault? No matter, somehow I would have to get through this. I thought long and hard about going someplace and having my baby and then giving it up for adoption, but the memories of my childhood and being raised by parents who did all the proper things but didn't quite love me were too strong. I'd been brought up a Catholic and knew the Church said abortion was wrong but I'd lapsed since I started college and just felt that the decision was mine to make, myself. Finally, I went to the school health service and spoke with a most compassionate nurse. She listened and laid out all my options. She said there were funds available for women like myself and she helped me make the arrangements for my abortion. It was early in the pregnancy so the procedure itself went easily and I didn't even have to be in the hospital. What hasn't been easy is forgiving myself and I've been in therapy for the two years since. Nothing has happened to my professor. He still teaches at the university and probably will until some girl has more courage than I did and turns him in.

B

Baby – an infant

    blue baby – an infant born with a bluish tint to the skin due to a congenital heart defect that allows the mixing of arterial and venous blood.

    baby blues – postnatal depression

    baby farms – 19th century facilities in which women gave birth, or to which newborns were sent, for the sole purpose of the infants being put up for adoption, often with a sizeable fee attached. Some operated completely outside of the law, others were quasi-legal.

Bacteremia – infection by bacteria in the bloodstream; usually accompanied by fever and malaise. If untreated may lead to septicemia and death. See **abortion, septic.**

Bactericidal – capable of killing bacteria.

Bacterium – a one-celled organism that has many biochemical properties, including the possibility of causing disease.

Bacteriuria – bacteria in the urine.

Bag of waters – popular name for the amniochorion (fetal membranes).

Bank – a place to collect and store organs, tissues or cells for future use.

    sperm bank – a place where sperm is frozen and stored for future use in artificial insemination.

Barren – popular term for sterile.

Barrett, James – retired Air Force Lt. Col. who, together with his wife June, a retired nurse, volunteered as clinic escorts at an abortion clinic in Pensacola, FL. He was murdered in 1994 by Paul Hill and June was severely injured. Also killed in that shooting was Dr. John Britton.

Barrett, June – a retired nurse who volunteered as a clinic escort with her husband, James. June was severely injured in the shooting in 1994 that left her husband and clinic doctor John Britton dead. The attack was perpetrated by Paul Hill.

Barrier – an obstruction or obstacle

    barrier contraception – utilizing a physical barrier, such as a condom or diaphragm, between the cervix and the sperm.

    placental barrier – the semi permeable layer of the placenta that separates the maternal and fetal circulation.

Bastardry – see illegitimacy

Battery – the touching of one person by another without consent.

    sexual battery – rape.

Baulieu, Dr Etienne-Emile – French researcher, part of team at the company Roussel Uclaf who developed the drug RU 486 (mifepristone) in the early 1980s, who was instrumental in organizing the first trials of the drug for medical abortion.

Bayliss, Dr – prosecuted for performing an abortion in Queensland, Australia, in 1985, he was acquitted. This was the last attempt to bring a doctor to court under Queensland's abortion laws.

Bearing down – the pushing effort made by a woman in the second stage of labor

Beat – pulsation, as in heart beat

Belgium – abortion legal and provided free of charge to Belgian citizens. After 12 weeks gestation abortion restricted to cases where the woman's health or life is endangered or severe fetal abnormality had been diagnosed. Belgium has one of the lowest rates of abortion in the world, around 6 per 1,000 women of reproductive age having an abortion each year. Belgian abortion rules require a 6 day **'cooling-off' period** between the time of a woman's first request for abortion and the performance of the procedure.

Belly – the abdomen

Belly button – the umbilicus or navel.

Belous, Leon – California doctor who was convicted in California in 1968 for referring women to an abortion clinic.

Benign – in speaking of a tumor, this means that it will not invade adjacent tissues nor will it metastasize (spread) to distant organs.

Beta-blocker – a drug that blocks certain nerves and is used to treat high blood pressure.

Betamethasone – a potent anti-inflammatory steroid, used as an oral or topical agent.

Bilirubin – a reddish-orange bile pigment formed from the breakdown of hemoglobin. An excess of bilirubin in the blood and tissues causes jaundice.

Bilirubinuria – the presence of bilirubin in the urine.

Bimanual exam – examination of the pelvis performed by a health provider who uses two fingers of one hand in the vagina and the other hand on the lower abdomen, enabling the pelvic organs to be felt between the examining hands.

Bioassay – evaluation of a substance by comparing its effects on a living organism or in-vitro preparation with a standard.

Biopsy – diagnostic procedure in which cells or tissue are removed in small amounts from a living body and examined.

Biorhythm – a biologically determined cyclic occurrence in a living organism.

Birth – the act of being born

  live birth – the complete expulsion or extraction of a fetus from the mother, regardless of the duration of pregnancy, following which the fetus gives evidence of life.

  premature birth – the birth of an infant after 20 weeks but before 37 weeks.

  stillbirth – the birth of an infant either premature or full term who after delivery does not breathe or show any other sign of life

Birth control – contraception. See methods under contraception.

Birth Control Review – early American publication providing a forum for the campaign to legalize and legitimate contraception.

Blastocyst – the embryo at the time of implantation into the inner wall of the uterus. It is comprised of a single outer layer of cells, a fluid-filled cavity, and an inner mass of cells. These are called the trophoblast, blastocele, and embryoblast, respectively.

Blastoma – malignant tumor of undifferentiated, embryonic cells.

Blastomere – one of the groups of cells into which the fertilized egg divides.

Bleeder – popular term for a person who has a bleeding disorder

Bleeding – loss of blood

Blood – the fluid circulated through the heart and blood vessels in a closed circuit. It consists of a pale yellow fluid called plasma in which are suspended both red and white blood cells and platelets.

  arterial blood – bright red blood that has been oxygenated in the lungs. This is the blood in the heart and arteries.

> **cord blood** – the blood within the umbilical cord. Important for stem cells.
>
> **occult blood** – microscopic quantities of blood.
>
> **venous blood** – dark red blood found in the veins. It has lost oxygen to the

tissues.

Blood bank – storage facility for blood for transfusion.

Blood group – genetically determined, immunological distinct classes of blood cells, determined by laboratory characteristics. Also known as blood type. Groups are A, B, O and AB.

Blood grouping – determining the group or type of blood by laboratory tests.

Blood type – see blood group

Blood typing – see blood grouping

Bonding – emotional attachment between mother and newborn in the perinatal period (immediately after birth).

Booth, Heather – American abortion rights activist who, together with other women activists, formed 'The Service' in Chicago. 'The Service' provided on-demand abortions to women and gained control over the quality and cost of abortions in the Chicago area. These activities were illegal at that time.

Bourne, Aleck – doctor who was prosecuted and acquitted in England in 1938 for performing an abortion on a fourteen-year-old rape victim. This case was implicit in later American challenges to abortion law and the effort to establish the need for legal therapeutic abortion.

Bowel – common name for the intestine.

bpas – see **British Pregnancy Advisory Service**

Brain – the portion of the central nervous system that is responsible for the coordination and control of all body activities. It is encased within the skull.

Bray, Michael – a Reformation Lutheran minister who is the spiritual father of the militant anti-abortion activists. He justifies violent acts against those involved in "killing the unborn." His website and his book 'A Time to Kill' inspired **Paul Hill**, among others.

Breach of duties – violation of responsibility owed to a patient to provide medical care within accepted standards of medical practice.

Breast cancer, risk of, following abortion – several studies have examined the relationship between abortion and the subsequent development of breast cancer. The largest and most comprehensive report on this subject appeared in the medical journal *The Lancet* in June 2004. The Collaborative Group on Hormonal Factors in Breast Cancer collected all the data from 53 separate studies carried out in 16 different countries, all with liberal abortion laws. The studies included 83,000 women who had been diagnosed with breast cancer, and they looked at the past histories of all these women – whether they had experienced an induced abortion, or a spontaneous miscarriage, or neither of these events. Studies were also divided into those where there was documented evidence of the abortion before the diagnosis of breast cancer was made, and those that depended on the woman's recall of her medical history. This was done to increase the accuracy of the information since women may vary in their willingness to report having an induced abortion in the past. The data were carefully analyzed and showed clearly that having either an induced abortion or a spontaneous miscarriage in the past did not increase a woman's chances of developing breast cancer in later life. This report is also known as the Beral report after the first author, Dr Valerie Beral. In addition a large Danish study involving 1.5 million women did not show any increase in risk of breast cancer in women who had undergone one or more previous abortions.

Breasts – the two glandular organs overlying the chest muscles. These organs make and provide milk for the infant. In the few days after birth and prior to milk being produced the breasts produce the fluid colostrum. Following late miscarriage or induced abortion (after 14 weeks) production of colostrum or milk may occur; this may be suppressed using drugs and with firm support of the breasts.

Breast-feeding – nursing the baby at the mother's breast.

Breech – buttocks.

breech presentation – buttocks presenting first at the birth canal.

British Pregnancy Advisory Service (bpas) – is a non-profit making charitable organization that is the largest specialist abortion provider in the United Kingdom outside the **NHS**, currently providing 27% of all abortions. bpas also provides comprehensive information about abortion and other options in unplanned pregnancy and contraceptive advice and services, In many areas bpas works in conjunction with NHS services to provide accessible abortion for women. bpas is also involved in education and research in the field of women's reproductive health.

Britton, John – a doctor at abortion clinic in Pensacola, FL. Murdered in July, 1994 by Paul Hill.

Broad spectrum – a term used to describe antibiotics active against a wide array of bacteria.

Buffer zones – around US abortion clinics, to protect clients and clinic personnel from picketing and threats to life and limb

C

Catherine

My partner Des and I were thrilled when I discovered that I was pregnant for the first time at age thirty-seven. I have been very successful in my career as a buyer for women's clothing chain and had delayed plans for pregnancy. Des and I had been trying to conceive for the past two years.

My pregnancy went along very well and I suffered none of the minor maladies that I had heard of from friends. I was just blooming with good health and the happiness of this pregnancy. At sixteen weeks, I had an amniocentesis to check for Down syndrome. Des and I had decided that this would be the responsible thing to do, after discussing various alternative options with our doctor.

As I watched the sonographer, Susan, run the ultrasound probe over my abdomen, prior to the insertion of the amniocentesis needle, I suddenly saw her expression change, and immediately felt an ominous premonition.

Susan summoned my obstetrician, who was just outside discussing another case with a radiologist. Together they all looked closely at the ultrasound images while I held Des's hand tight, unable to speak a word. Then Dr Nguyen and Susan almost imperceptibly shook their heads. Dr. Nyugen turned to me and gently explained to me that the amniocentesis would be unnecessary: my ultrasound clearly showed that our fetus had multiple abnormalities. Our baby had no kidneys, facial deformities and his heart had not properly developed. These abnormalities were incompatible with life. If we wished to do so, medical abortion could be carried out.

We asked for some time alone together. We cried together and resolved that we had no choice but to agree to the therapeutic abortion. Dr Nguyen then sat down and explained the procedure of medical abortion to both of us. We decided to delay the procedure until Des could have time off work to stay with me.

Two agonizing days later, on the same floor of the same hospital where I had planned an all-natural birth of a beautiful baby, I had misoprostol tablets inserted vaginally over a six-hour period. Contractions began for which I was given Stadol and Des sat and held my hand throughout. In a further six hours, I delivered our tiny son. He neither breathed nor cried. We held him and named him Nathaniel. The nurses took photos and footprints for a memory book and then we arranged with the chaplain for a simple burial.

Eighteen months later, I gave birth in the same hospital to our healthy daughter, Natasha.

C

California – the California Senate and House are both pro-choice. The state received an A+ rating for access from **NARAL**. Performance of abortion is legally restricted to physicians. Any healthcare worker who registers in writing an objection to abortion on moral, ethical or religious grounds is allowed to legally refuse to provide abortion services. There exists a California law prohibiting abortion to a minor without prior parental consent or judicial authorization, but this law has been held unconstitutional by the California Supreme Court because it violates the explicit right of privacy set forth in the California Constitution. California has specific requirements for 'information and education sessions' to inform the woman about how the abortion is performed, possible risks and complications, and alternatives to abortion. California law also provides that abortion may be performed on a viable fetus only when continuation of the pregnancy poses a risk to the health of the pregnant woman in the good faith judgment of her physician. California law explicitly allows pharmacists to provide emergency contraception to women without a prescription according to a specific protocol, which includes the provision to the woman of a fact sheet telling her how to use the product, when to seek medical follow-up and all other necessary information. California law guarantees that women's prescriptions for contraceptives will be filled. It also requires that all insurance plans that cover prescription drugs also cover contraception. California state law affirms a woman's right to choose and to privacy in her reproductive choices. The California Constitution defines reproductive choice as a fundamental right. Women who qualify for state medical assistance are able to obtain abortions paid for by these state funds. Abortion providers and clinics are protected by law from blockades and violence.

Calderone, Mary S – medical director of Planned Parenthood in the US in 1955. Played a crucial role in spurring a professional movement to reexamine and reform the abortion laws in America.

Campaign Life Coalition – a pro-life organization in Canada.

Canada – abortion is not limited by law in Canada. It was banned in 1869, and in 1892 abortion and the advertisement and dispensing of contraception were made illegal. Illegal abortion flourished and led to many deaths. In 1969, a law was passed that provided for legal abortion when a three-doctor committee determined that the health of the woman was endangered. The same bill also legalized homosexuality and contraception, but did not remove abortion from the Criminal Code. In 1973, **Henry Morgentaler**, a Montreal physician, made a public statement that he had performed abortions without going before the required committee. He was tried and repeatedly (through appeals) found not guilty. The Quebec government declared the abortion law unenforceable as a result. Over the next 15 years Morgentaler challenged the law in other provinces and in 1988 the Supreme Court of Canada found the abortion law to be unconstitutional. It found that the law breached the woman's right to security of her person, a right which is guaranteed in Canada's Charter of Rights and Freedoms. Since this time, no new law has been successfully passed. In another case before the Supreme Court, Tremblay v. Daigle, it was ruled that only the woman has choice in the matter of abortion; the father has no legal say. The courts have also determined that the fetus does not have rights independent of the mother in whose body it resides.

As it stands, abortion is available on demand and is paid for by public funds through the Canadian Medicare system. Medical abortion utilizing **methotrexate** and **misoprostol** is available in a limited fashion; mifepristone is not available and cannot be legally imported. In 2002, 15.4 of every 1000 Canadian women had an abortion. Politically, abortion is considered to be a low priority issue for most Canadians.

Canadian Federation for Sexual Health – affiliate of Planned Parenthood International, this organization counsels and refers women for abortion but does not engage in political lobbying.

Canal – a tubular structure or channel.

       birth canal – canal through which the fetus passes in birth. It consists of the dilated cervical opening, the vagina and vulva. Also called parturient or obstetrical canal.

Cancer, of breast – see breast cancer

Cancer, of uterus – see uterine cancer

Candida – a yeast-like fungus

       C. albicans – a species that normally inhabits the gastrointestinal tract but that can cause infection in the vagina, mouth or throat in certain conditions, such as pregnancy, diabetes, or immune disorders. Also called thrush.

Cannula – long plastic tube used to aspirate or extract material from the uterine cavity by vaccum or manual means

Cap – any device that resembles or serves as a cover.

       cervical cap – a small contraceptive device that fits over the cervix. This is designed to prevent pregnancy. Also known as the contraceptive cap or vault.

Caput – head; also the soft edematous tissue normally present on the head of a newborn infant resulting from the normal physical pressures of the birth

Carrier – an individual who carries an abnormal gene that has not manifested in that individual but that can be transmitted to children born to that person. These recessive genes can be detected by DNA testing.

Carter, Patricia A. – physician author of a 1944 article calling for limitation of the practice of therapeutic abortion to those cases in which the mother's life is in imminent danger.

Cartilage – the firm, somewhat elastic connective tissue that constitutes the major part of the fetal skeleton. It is also present in the adult nose, ear, auditory canal, larynx, trachea and bronchi.

Castrate – to remove the ovaries or testes surgically.

Catherwood, Albert E. – reported in 1939 on the formation of a 'permanent therapeutic abortion committee' at a Detroit, Michigan hospital. In addition to deciding whether a particular therapeutic abortion should be performed, this committee also considered whether sterilizations should be performed. It is probably the first such committee formed in the US.

Catheter – a slender, usually flexible tube that is inserted into a body cavity for the purpose of introducing a substance or draining substances, e.g. urine, or for performing procedures. Catheters were used to induce abortion in earlier years. A rubber catheter was inserted into the cervical os, irritating the cervix and causing contractions and abortion.

These were used by early physician and midwife abortionists.

Catheterization – introduction of a catheter into a body cavity for therapeutic purposes (e.g. to drain urine) or to obtain information for diagnosis.

Catholic Church – officially opposes abortion for any reason. However, an *amici* brief was filed in the case of Webster v. Reproductive Health Services, 1989, by Catholics for a Free Choice, Chicago Catholic Women, and the National Coalition of American Nuns in which they hold that there is no constant teaching in the Catholic Church on the beginning of personhood and the infusion of the physical with the soul. According to the teachings of Aquinas, the early fetus is not ensouled and therefore, is not a person. In the Church, from 1140 through 1869, church law distinguished between the unensouled and the ensouled fetus as regards the gravity of abortion and any guilt thereby attached. Vatican II expressly avoided defining the point of ensoulment. The authors of the brief point out that there is no consistent tradition in regard to abortion and that in all matters, Catholic theology holds that the informed conscience of the individual must rule.

Catholic rates of abortion – rate is approximately 24 abortions per 1000 pregnancies in Catholic women in the United States.

Cauda equina – a group of nerves extending beyond the end of the spinal cord and occupying the lower third of the vertebral canal. These nerves originate from the lumbar, sacral and coccygeal segments of the spinal cord.

Caul – the portion of the fetal membranes that may surround the head of the baby at birth.

Cauterization – the searing of body tissues by heat, electricity or chemicals to stop bleeding or promote healing.

CDC – see **Centers for Disease Control**

Cell – the smallest unit of life – i.e. the smallest unit of any living organism that is capable of functioning independently.

> **germ cell** – an ovum or spermatocyte. A cell containing the reproductive material of either male or female; a germinal cell; reproductive cell.

Cellulitis – a rapidly spreading infection of subcutaneous tissue occurring as a complication of a wound infection.

> **pelvic cellulitis** – see parametritis

Centers for Disease Control – a US federal agency responsible for US programs of prevention and control of communicable diseases. It is also responsible for environmental health issues. In an outbreak of disease, it is responsible for directing quarantine and advising the public health response. In addition, it conducts epidemiological research.

Cephalic – referring to the head.

Cephalization – growth of the structures and functions of the head in the embryo.

Cephalomegaly – abnormal enlargement of the head.

Cephalometry – measurement of the head.

> **ultrasonic cephalometry** – measurement of the head by ultrasound.

Cephalosporins – a commonly used class of antibiotics.

Cerclage – a surgical placement of a suture in the cervix in an attempt to prevent miscarriage.

Cerebrospinal – relates to brain and spinal cord.

Cervical – relating to the uterine cervix

Cervical incompetence – failure of the cervix to remain closed during pregnancy, leading to miscarriage or premature birth. May be caused by excessive or forced mechanical dilatation of the cervix during abortion of a previous pregnancy. Can be treated by inserting a stitch encircling the cervix at around 14 weeks of pregnancy. Cervical damage during surgical abortion is minimized by the use of medical methods of **cervical ripening**.

Cervical priming – see cervical ripening.

Cervical ripening – the changes that occur in the cervix as it prepares for the first stage of childbirth. Cervical ripening can also be induced artificially using the drug misoprostol, prior to performing surgical abortion.

Cervicitis – inflammation of the cervix of the uterus, often caused by a sexually transmitted disease, such as Chlamydia or gonorrhea.

Cervix – any neck-like part of an organ or structure, most commonly used in relation to the uterus (womb.).

> **double** – a developmental anomaly resulting in two uterine cervixes in a woman.
> **incompetent** – a cervix that is prone to dilate prematurely in pregnancy, usually resulting in miscarriage or premature delivery.
> **ripe** – popular term for the softening of the cervix in reparation for labor.
> **uterine** – the neck of the uterus.

Cesarean section – delivery of a baby through an incision made through the abdominal and uterine walls.

Chancre – an ulcer formed at the site of penetration of the organism (*Treponema pallidum*) causing syphilis. Also called 'hard chancre.'

Chancroid – a sexually transmitted disease caused by *Hemophilus ducreyi*. It is characterized by one or more soft, painful ulcers on the genitalia.

Change – a modification.

Children by Choice – Australian organization based in Queensland that aims to give unbiased information to women with unplanned pregnancies. Information on abortion, adoption and parenting is provided.

Childbirth – the process of giving birth to a child.

China – legal access to early abortion, both medical and surgical, is easy and China's maternal mortality rate is low.

Chlamydia – bacterial group, some of which are sexually transmitted and cause infection in the genitourinary tract and possible infertility. These infections can also be transmitted to the newborn during birth.

Chorion – the cellular, outermost membrane enveloping the fetus.

Christian Heritage Party of Canada – Canada's only declared pro-life federal political party.

Chromosome – a group of threadlike structures within the nucleus of a cell. These structures contain DNA and encode the genetic information of the cell. Human cells normally contain 46 chromosomes.

> **Sex chromosomes** – chromosomes involved in determining the gender of an individual. These are designated X and Y and a female has XX and a male XY.

Clavicle – the long curved bone extending from the breastbone to the shoulder.

Clergy Consultation Service (New York) – a joint Protestant-Jewish service active prior to legalization of abortion – counseled women seeking abortions before and after their procedures, supported movement for safe legal abortion.

Clidotomy – surgical division of the clavicles of a dead fetus to make delivery easier for the mother.

Clinic – a facility where medical care is given to patients who do not require hospitalization.

Clinical – relating to the observation of the symptoms, signs and course of an illness.

Clostridium sordellii – bacteria which can live normally in the bowel and rectal areas of the body, in both women and men, without causing any harm – this is called 'colonization.' Many other bacteria similarly live in these areas. Occasionally following childbirth or surgery (cesarean, gynaecologic surgery, bowel or bone surgery) these bacteria can infect the wound or the interior of the uterus; in this situation the bacteria can produce a powerful toxin which may be rapidly fatal. Deaths from *Clostridium sordellii* infection have been reported rarely in the United States following normal vaginal births, caesarean section, abdominal and orthopaedic surgery.

From September 2000 when mifepristone was approved for use in the United States until June 2005, there were four reported deaths associated with mifepristone/vaginal misoprostol use for medical abortion. All of these deaths occurred in California. The deaths were all preceded by an illness characterized by low blood pressure and a rapid pulse but no fever. There was abdominal pain, vomiting and diarrhea. Subsequent to investigations overseen by the **FDA** and **CDC** *Clostridium sordellii* was demonstrated as the cause of death in all four cases. Investigation failed to show any contamination of either the mifepristone or the misoprostol used, or any link to the techniques of medical abortion used. The FDA is also aware of a further case of fatal *Clostridium* sepsis which occurred in Canada in 2001. No cases of *Clostridium* infection have been reported in association with medical abortion in countries outside North America. Aware of the public interest and concern about this matter, the FDA has maintained a Questions and Answers section about *Clostridium sordellii* on its website www.fda.gov/cder/drug/infopage/mifepristone

Coitus – vaginal sexual intercourse between a man and woman.

College women – in the Kinsey Study, college educated women tended to abort a greater proportion of pregnancies during the college years and bear children later. Women with only an elementary education bore more children and had more abortions than women with greater levels of education.

Colorado – D rated by **NARAL**. Legislature is pro-choice. Colorado has not repealed its pre-Roe ban on abortion. Only physicians may perform abortions in Colorado. A married woman is required by law to obtain her husband's consent before having an abortion; this law has been deemed unconstitutional by the US Supreme Court. Colorado restricts state funding for abortion except in cases of rape, incest or life-endangering condition. This applies to low-income women relying on state medical assistance plans and to state employees whose insurance plans do not cover abortion services. Any person employed by a hospital may be excused from participation in medical procedures that result in abortion if they file a written refusal based on moral or religious grounds. Colorado law requires notification of both parents of a minor woman 48 hours prior to her having an abortion. No exception is made for victims of rape or incest. It may be waived only on grounds of reported child abuse and in the case of a life-threatening emergency. Colorado law does protect people seeking reproductive health care from blockade and violence.

Colostrum – sticky yellowish fluid produced by the breasts in late pregnancy and the first few days after delivery.

Common law – under common law, abortion in America was legal until 'quickening' defined as the time at which a woman could feel fetal movement [around the fourth month 4 of pregnancy.] This was tacitly accepted in colonial America and was specifically confirmed in court in Massachusetts in 1812. The legal basis for this position was traditional British common law.

Comstock Act – 1873 'Act for the Suppression of Trade in and Circulation of Obscene Literature and Articles of Immoral Use.' This law was designed to curtail the proliferation of pornography and the trade of information, medicines, and articles designed to be used to cause abortion, except when prescribed by a physician in good standing.

Comstock, Anthony – leader of the anti-obscenity movement in the 1870s. He was the head of the New York Society for the Suppression of Vice and spearheaded the passage of the law that bore his name. Under the 1873 Comstock Act, Comstock became a special agent of the federal government, empowered with enforcement of the Act. As such, he became an aggressive prosecutor of abortionists

Conception – the fertilization of an ovum by a sperm.

    wrongful conception – a term of medical negligence in which pregnancy results from a physician's failure to inform parents that 1) a sterilization procedure might be unsuccessful or 2) a genetic risk present may result in a defective fetus.

Conceptus – all the tissue products of conception from the time of fertilization until birth; it includes the placenta, membranes, and the embryo/fetus.

Condom – a sheath placed over the erect penis before intercourse to form a barrier between the sperm and the cervical canal. This is usually made of latex or plastic and also serves to protect against sexually transmitted diseases. Condoms made from natural membranes do not protect against disease.

    female condom – a sheath that is worn in the vagina to give the same protections as the male condom. Most varieties have a closed inner end and an outer flexible ring to hold the condom in place.

Condyloma – a wart. Caused by human papilloma virus (HPV). Most are benign, but some strains of HPV are associated with cervical cancer.

Congenital – present at birth.

Connecticut – A rated by **NARAL**. Legislature is pro-choice. Only physicians are allowed to perform abortions. This law was amended to allow licensed nurse-practitioners, nurse-midwives, and physician's assistants to prescribe mifepristone under a physician's supervision. Connecticut law imposes certain regulations on abortion providers that are not imposed on other healthcare providers. These are: all outpatient clinics providing abortion services, regardless of procedures offered, are required to have a standard operating room, all clinics must hire counselors who have or are supervised by a person with credentials in psychology, nursing, counseling, social work, or ministry, and all abortions after the second trimester must be performed in hospital. Connecticut has an abortion-specific informed consent law and requires women younger than 16 to receive counseling prior to having an abortion. Connecticut prohibits abortion on a viable fetus. Connecticut law upholds the right to reproductive choice and its constitution provides greater protection for reproductive choice than does the US Constitution. Low-income women who qualify for state medical assistance have access to abortion paid for by state funds. Any insurance plan offering prescription drug coverage must provide the same coverage for contraception. People seeking reproductive healthcare are protected by law from blockade or violence.

Consanguineous – genetically related.

Consanguinity – blood relationship

Conscientious objection – rights of medical personnel and/or paramedical personnel to exclude themselves from a medical procedure e.g. abortion on religious or ethical grounds. Incorporated into law in many countries and states – usually with the requirement that the objection be tendered in writing

Consent – voluntary agreement to medical care or treatment by one with the mental capacity to do so, or in the case of a minor or incapacitated person, their legal representative.

    informed consent – voluntary permission as above based on a full and frank discussion of the benefits of the treatment, the risks involved, the possible complications and adverse effects, alternative methods of treatment and the consequences of denying such permission.

Consenting adolescent – also known as the 'Mature Minor' doctrine. Although the age of majority is 18 in most US states, most states permit adolescents to consent for pelvic exams, screening and treatment of STDs, contraception, prenatal care, examination and treatment following sexual assault, diagnosis and treatment of substance abuse, and assessment and treatment of mental health disorders. The adolescent has the right to privacy in these settings.

Contraception – the use of drugs, chemicals, devices, methods or procedures to prevent conception.

    barrier contraception – placing a physical barrier, such as a condom, between the sperm and the cervical canal and thereby preventing fertilization. Includes condoms, diaphragms, and cervical caps.

    chemical contraception – anything containing a spermicidal substance that is introduced into the vagina prior to intercourse. This includes foams, gels, suppositories, sponges and creams.

    emergency contraception – also referred to as post-coital contraception -term covering a number of different medications which may be taken within a given time period following unprotected sexual intercourse. Unprotected intercourse may be that for which contraception was not used, or was used and is thought to have failed e.g. tears in condoms or diaphragms. Emergency contraception may also be indicated following intercourse where relatively ineffective contraceptive methods were used e.g. spermicide alone. The medications used for emergency contraception have a high rate of success in preventing implantation and continuing pregnancy but none is 100% effective. In some countries these meds can be bought over the counter from pharmacists, in others a doctor's prescription is required. Currently used emergency contraceptives include:

levonorgestrel – marketed in the US as Plan-B, in Australia as Postinor and Nolevho, in the UK as Levonelle. This synthetic progestagen is taken in two doses of $750\mu g$, the first within 72 hours of unprotected intercourse, the second twelve hours later. The sooner the medication is taken following unprotected intercourse the more effective it is likely to be. Levonorgestrel will not terminate an implanted pregnancy nor will it damage the embryo if unprotected intercourse has occurred earlier in the cycle and pregnancy resulted.

Levonorgestrel acts by altering the endometrium making it less receptive to a fertilized ovum; it also may act to delay ovulation. Since the introduction of Plan B in the US, there has been a reduction in the number of abortions nationwide.

The **Yuzpe** method- uses two tablets of one of the older types of the oral contraceptive pill taken together (containing in total 100μg ethinyl estradiol and 0.5 mg levonorgestrel) followed by a second similar dose 12 hours later. Must be taken within 72 hours of unprotected sex. Failure rate is 2-3%. Nausea and vomiting are common side effects which is why the levonorgestrel regimen, which does not have such effects, has become more widely used.

Copper-releasing **intrauterine devices** can be effective emergency contraceptive measures if placed within 120 hours of unprotected intercourse and also serve for ongoing contraception.

Mifepristone (RU 486) has been successfully used as emergency contraception in smaller doses than that required for medical abortion, but is not generally available in most countries. It is effective up to 5 days following unprotected sex; side effects are minimal but the next menstrual period may be delayed.

hormonal contraception – any oral, injected, transdermal or transvaginal administration of synthetic steroids on a regular dose schedule to prevent conception. This includes the Pill, the patch, the ring and the combination hormone shot and Depo shot.

intrauterine device, as contraception – a device (Copper T, Mirena) introduced into the uerus to prevent pregnancy from developing.

Contraceptive – anything that prevents conception.

'Cooling-off period' – term used to describe the compulsory waiting period between a woman's first requesting an abortion and the performance of the procedure; this is a requirement in many US states, European countries and other jurisdictions.

Cosgrove, Samuel A. – physician co-author, with Patricia A. Carter, of 1944 article calling for stringent control of therapeutic abortion.

Counseling – professional guidance in psychosocial situations, intended to give a person an understanding of her problems, and potentialities and alternatives. In many US states and other jurisdictions pre-abortion counseling is mandatory.

Craniotomy – procedure in which the head of a fetus is punctured and its contents evacuated to allow a vaginal delivery; this is performed to allow the delivery of a dead fetus or in **partial-birth abortion.**

Curette – a tubular instrument with a spoon-shaped tip for scraping the inner wall or lining of a body cavity.

Curettage – the removal of tissue from the inner wall of a cavity with a spoon-shaped instrument. This may be used to remove abnormal tissue, for diagnostic purposes, following miscarriage or during surgical abortion.

endometrial curettage – scraping of the interior lining of the uterus with a sharp-edged curette.

suction curettage (vacuum aspiration) – removal of or sampling of uterine contents by using a suction curette.

Cystitis – inflammation or infection of the urinary bladder.

D

Donna

I'm a lawyer and being a woman in a man's world, you just have to be better than they are. If your colleague works seventy hours a week, you have to work ninety. If he plays golf with the senior partner, well, you have to find ways to make that partner feel like the most important man in the world. But not by going to bed with him, oh no, that's a surefire way to screw up your career. Pun intended. I always have to look like my hair was just done, my clothes fresh from the dry cleaners and make up is perfectly applied. All my male colleagues have to do is shine their shoes and wear a tie.

There's not much time for social life with my work. Maybe that's why I fell into a comfortable, but not exciting, relationship with Bernie, aka Bernard Towson Tyler, III. Bernie is a nice guy and being with him helps my career because he's old family money and my boss likes that, but he doesn't exactly rock my world. We've lived together now for five years and I suppose if there was a good reason, we'd get married. But there is none.

Things went along like that for about three years and then suddenly, I found myself pregnant. I was thirty-three and had never been pregnant before. I had an IUD in and had always been very careful anyway. Bernie and I didn't use condoms anymore, but I never thought I'd get pregnant. There was no room in my life for children; I had never wanted to be a mother and I still don't. I'm not the motherly type. So I went ahead and had a medical termination. For some reason, it didn't seem to be any of Bernie's business so I didn't tell him before I went. One night it slipped out and he was furious. He accused me of killing his baby and of treating him like a cypher. And then, he just walked out of the apartment and stayed away for a week. No calls, nothing. I felt bad about that and I could see how he'd been hurt by my actions and I was sorry about that part of it, so I tracked him down and we had a long talk.
I'm not sorry about having the abortion. I would not be a good mother; I'm too selfish and too career-driven. Bernie and I agreed that I'd have my tubes tied and if he decides that he wants the whole family scene sometime in the future, we'll have an amicable parting of the ways. For now, we're pretty good together and it is easy.

D

D & C – see Dilatation and curettage

D & E – see dilatation and evacuation.

Davidson, Dr – medical practitioner against whom prosecution was attempted in 1969 in Melbourne, Australia. The decision by Justice Menhennitt in this case defined the conditions in which abortion could be lawfully performed in Victoria.

Del-M – a device used to perform menstrual extraction. It consists of a cannula inserted into the stopper of a collection jar. The suction is provided by a syringe connected by a one-way valve through the stopper of the collection jar.

Demographics – vital statistics. For 2002, the rate of abortion in the US was estimated by the Alan Guttmacher Institute to be 20.9 or 20.9 women of every 1000 women aged 15 – 44 years had an abortion in 2002. The ratio of abortions to every 100 live births in 2002 was 24.2.

The majority of women obtaining abortions in US are white (~70% in 1973, ~59% in 1999) but rates are highest among black and Hispanic women. Black women at or above 200% poverty had abortion rates 2-3 times those of Hispanic women and 3-4 times those of non-Hispanic whites.

More than 80% of women having abortions are unmarried.

Since 1980, the majority of women having abortions are already mothers.

Almost 90% of abortions are performed in the first trimester.

2000 statistics USA: 1.31 million abortions.

    2.1 % women aged 15 -44 had abortion.

    57.6% aborted at < 9 weeks, 20.3% at 9–10 weeks, 10.2% at 11–12 weeks, 6.2% at 13–15 weeks, 4.3% at 16–20 weeks, and 1.5% at 20+ weeks

    Risk of death: 0.6 deaths per 100,000 abortions

    Risk of major complications: < 1%

    Age of woman at time of abortion:

        <15 yrs – 0.7%

        15 -19 – 18.6%

        20 -24 –33%

        25-29 – 23.1%

        30-34 – 13.5%

        35-39 – 8.1%

        40-44 – 3.1%

    Religious affiliation, in the USA: abortion rate for Protestants: 17 per 1000 pregnancies; Catholics: 24 per 1000 pregnancies. Women with no religious affiliation have highest abortion rates at 30 per 1000 pregnancies. Of total abortions, Protestant women comprise 37% and Catholic women, 31%.

Depo Provera – injectable contraceptive consisting of the synthetic progestin (progestagen), medroxyprogesterone acetate. One injection of 150 mg is given every three months.

Depression – morbid sadness and lack of interest in one's surroundings, accompanied by lack of energy, may range from mild to severe.

      endogenous depression – occurring without external triggers.

      depression following induced abortion – see psychological effects of induced abortion

      major depression – depressive disorder including at least four of the following, occurring daily for at least two weeks:1) recurrent suicidal ideation, with or without attempts, 2) change in appetite, with corresponding weight change, 3) insomnia or excessive sleeping, 4) loss of interest and pleasure in daily life and decreased libido, 5) feelings of worthlessness, self-reproach and excessive guilt, 6) sluggishness or agitation, 7) difficulty in making decisions, and 8) fatigue. This is a serious and disabling condition.

      postpartum depression – a mood disorder experienced by some women in the time after delivery. Most common is a temporary phase of feeling weepy, irritable, forgetful and experiencing mood swings in the time soon after giving birth. It can however be a major depressive illness, as characterized above, in which case the mother can be a danger to both herself and her baby, and early and appropriate medical intervention is necessary.

Depression, period 1929-1939 – Social and economic conditions in the Depression played an important role in bringing the needs of women for safe legal abortion to the attention of physicians.

Device – anything constructed for a specific purpose.

      contraceptive device – any device for preventing conception.

      intrauterine device – a device made of plastic or metal, treated or not with a hormone or other drug, that can be inserted into the uterus to prevent conception.

Diaphragm – a dome-shaped rubber disc that is inserted into the vagina prior to sexual intercourse to cover the cervix, forming a seal between the sperm and the cervical canal and thus preventing pregnancy. Prior to each use, the diaphragm is coated with a spermicidal cream or gel to improve its efficacy.

Dilatation (dilation) – the condition of being stretched or enlarged.

Dilatation and curettage (D&C) – stretching of the uterine cervix and scraping of the lining of the uterus, either by a curette or by a vacuum aspirator, up to 14 weeks' gestation..

Dilatation and evacuation (D&E) – induced abortion after 16 weeks gestation, produced by widely dilating the cervix followed by mechanically destroying and removing fetal parts, followed by vacuum aspiration of remaining uterine contents. D&E should only be performed in a suitable clinic or hospital setting by a fully trained and experienced operator.

Dilate – to stretch.

Dilator – instrument for enlarging a passage, cavity or opening. In performing a surgical abortion, dilatation is first carried out using steel dilators of increasing size to gradually enlarge the width of the cervical canal so that extraction of the pregnancy can then take place. Dilatation of the cervix may be assisted by the prior use of drugs such as **misoprostol** or devices such as **laminaria tents** – use of one or other of these may cause sufficient softening and opening of the canal to remove the need for instrumental dilatation altogether. Cervical dilatation should be performed by a health professional with appropriate training and experience as there is a risk of immediate damage of the cervix and adjacent organs, and of long-term damage causing **cervical incompetence**

with late miscarriage or premature birth in subsequent pregnancies.

District of Columbia – rated B- by **NARAL.** Performance of abortion is restricted to physicians. Any individual may refuse to participate in direct patient care that conflicts with his or her religious or ethical beliefs; such individuals must notify immediate supervisors in writing of their conflict prior to any assignment in conflict with their beliefs. Any employee is required to provide for patient safety and avoid abandonment. The District of Columbia prohibits public funding for abortion unless the procedure is necessary to preserve the life of the mother or when the pregnancy is the result of rape or incest. The District of Columbia provides protection against clinic and provider blockades and violence. .

Dose – a specified amount of drug given at stated times or intervals.

   effective dose – the amount of a drug necessary to produce the desired effect.

Douching – washing the vagina by a spray of a variety of liquids, usually after intercourse to remove the ejaculate or after menses as a cleansing. Early attempt at contraception –douching is not an effective method of contraception.

Downer, Carol – inventor, together with Lorraine Rothman, of the Del-M device.

Drink Safe strips – test strips and coasters that are designed to change color when moistened with a drink containing gamma hydroxybutyrate or Rohypnol, date rape drugs. These were brought on the market in 2002 and are small enough to easily fit in a woman's purse.

Drug – any chemical capable of affecting living processes.

Dysmelia – congenital absence of one or more extremities, in part or whole.

Dysmorphism – abnormalities of shape, as seen in various genetic or environmentally caused syndromes.

Dysontogenesis – abnormal development.

Dyspareunia – painful sexual intercourse.

Dystocia – difficult labor.

E

Elisa

I got pregnant when I was eighteen. My baby's father was long out of the picture; we broke up after two or three dates. My parents were a great help in taking care of me during my pregnancy and with Marnie after she was born. It was a difficult pregnancy. My blood pressure went sky high and I was in and out of the hospital. At thirty-six weeks, I had a seizure and Marnie was born early, by C-section. She had to stay in the hospital for a couple of weeks after I was able to go home, but she has been healthy and was even early with walking and talking, so I was happy. When Marnie was four, I decided to go back to school. I wanted to start an interior design business someday.

During the first month of attending classes at the community college, I met Scott. It was a whirlwind romance and we married eighteen months later. Marnie was our flower girl. I guess I'm one of those tremendously fertile women, because I got pregnant with Jamie right away. It was another roller coaster pregnancy and I spent a lot of time in the hospital. This time I didn't end up with convulsions, but they took Jamie by cesarean a few weeks before his due date. I went on the minipill but I guess I must have missed one or two during those sleepless nights with a little baby, because when Jamie was four months old I was pregnant again.

We were aghast and Scott and I went right away to see Dr. McGee. He explained to us that we were correct in being alarmed, that it was very risky for me to be pregnant again at all and especially so soon. My blood pressure was still high and I was tired a lot. Besides the physical risk to me, he was concerned that it would be a great emotional burden to have a high risk pregnancy while caring for a newborn and an older child, as well as going to school and working. Dr. McGee said that he rarely makes such a recommendation, but he thought it would be in our best interest for me to have a surgical abortion and a tubal ligation at the same time. We agreed but it was not an easy decision, although neither of us is religious. But we believe now, five years later, that we made the right decision and have always been very grateful to have our two healthy children and for me to have regained my health.

E

EC – see Emergency contraception.

Eclampsia – an acute disorder occurring in women during or just after pregnancy and associated with high blood pressure. It is characterized by seizures, often occurring without warning, and is life-threatening.

Ectopic pregnancy – pregnancy developing outside the cavity of the uterus, usually in one or other fallopian tube. As the pregnancy develops it stretches the narrow tube which may rupture with severe internal bleeding that is potentially fatal for the woman. Whenever early pregnancy is diagnosed the physician should be alert for the possibility of ectopic pregnancy; about 19 pregnancies per 1000 are ectopic. If abortion, surgical or medical, is attempted and ectopic pregnancy is not recognized the tube may subsequently rupture causing maternal death. Treatment of diagnosed ectopic pregnancy is usually by surgery, either using the laparoscope or an open surgery depending on the urgency of the case. **Methotrexate** is sometimes used to treat early ectopic pregnancy but **mifepristone** is not effective for this purpose; when methotrexate is used the woman must be under close medical supervision.

Ectrodactyly – congenital absence of fingers and toes.

Ectromelia – congenital absence of one or more limbs.

Edema – soft tissue swelling due to fluid accumulated in the intercellular spaces.

Education, effect on abortion – statistics for the US from year 2000:, among women 20 and older: at least some college education – 57% of all abortions done (with an abortion rate of 26 per 1000 pregnancies); high school graduates – 30% of abortions; less than high school graduation – 13% of abortions. Statistics are from 2000 – 2001. College graduates have an abortion rate of 13 per 1000 pregnancies and have shown a higher than average decline in abortion rates (30%) since 1994.

Egg – see ovum.

    fertilized egg – see zygote

Ejaculate – to suddenly discharge, especially semen.

Ejaculation – the discharge of semen from the urethra during orgasm.

Elective – non-urgent.

Embolism – blockage of a blood vessel by a clot or other solid or gaseous mass that has been transported by the bloodstream to the point of blockage.

    amniotic fluid embolism – rare complication of labor in which amniotic fluid enters the mother's circulation and causes hemorrhage, shock and pulmonary embolus.

    pulmonary embolism – blockage of one of the blood vessels in the lungs. This occurs as a complication of childbirth or surgery and in patients who are immobilized for any reason. It is also an uncommon complication of hormonal contraception.

Embolus – plug or blockage within a blood vessel that is carried by the blood flow to a remote site.

Embryo – an organism in its earliest stage of development; in humans, from conception until the end of the eighth week.

Embryology – the study of living organisms from conception until birth.

Emergency contraception – see **Contraceptives, emergency,** formerly referred to as the 'morning-after' pill.

Emmenogogic – inducing menstrual flow. Usually applied to drugs or herbs, often toxic, used to try to induce abortion prior to the liberalization of abortion laws.

Emmenogogue – any agent inducing menstruation.

Endometrial – referring to the lining of the uterus.

Endometriosis – a disorder in which abnormal tissue growth, microscopically like endometrial tissue, is found in locations outside of the interior of the uterus. It can cause pain and infertility.

Endometritis – inflammation of the lining of the uterus.

Endometrium – the secretory mucous membrane lining of the interior of the uterus.

Endoscope – a tubular telescope-like instrument with a light source for viewing the interior of a hollow organ, such as the uterus.

Endoscopy – inspection of a body cavity or organ through an endoscope.

Engorgement – the condition of being distended due to an excess accumulation of fluid.

> **breast engorgement** – accumulation of lymph and venous blood in breast tissue, occurring in the breasts in the first post-partum week. Also used for breasts distended with milk in breastfeeding mothers.

Episiotomy – incision of the perineum for a controlled enlargement of the vaginal opening at the time of emergence of the presenting part of the baby from the birth canal. Performed primarily to prevent imminent tears or to prevent undue pressure on the fetal skull in premature birth.

Ergonovine – drug which brings about a sustained contraction of the uterus. Used extensively in midwifery and obstetrics to prevent bleeding after childbirth; also useful to prevent or treat heavy bleeding associated with miscarriage or induced abortion In the UK and other countries known as ergometrine.

Estradiol – Estrogenic female hormone from the ovaries and placenta. It is essential for the development and proper functioning of the female reproductive organs and prepares the endometrium for the implantation of the fertilized ovum.

> **ethinyl estradiol** – a semi synthetic form used in many oral contraceptives.

Estriol – relatively weak estrogenic hormone; also a metabolic product of the hormones estradiol and estrone. Especially abundant in the urine of pregnant women.

Estrogen – general term for the group of female sex hormones.

Estrone – estrogenic hormone found in the ovaries.

Ethical – in conformity with professionally accepted principles.

Ethics – standards of conduct governing an individual or profession.

Evacuation – the process of emptying or removing.

Evaluation – examination and judgment of the significance of something.

Examination – an investigation for the purpose of making a diagnosis or evaluating treatment.

> **bimanual pelvic examination** – an examination conducted using the index and middle fingers of one hand of the examiner placed within the vagina, and the flat surface of the other hand on the lower abdominal wall, in order to feel structures, such as the uterus and ovaries, between the two examining hands.

Extraction – the act of moving or drawing out, such as the removal of a fetus from the birth canal, either manually or with instruments.

menstrual extraction – see **aspiration, menstrual**.

Extractor – any instrument or device used in pulling out.

Extrauterine – outside the uterus.

Extremity – an arm or leg.

F

Francesca

Mother was born in 1913 and married my father just as World War II broke out. After the war, they settled in Los Angeles and my mother was forced to work as a domestic since all aircraft and government jobs were turned over to men returning from the War. My father briefly drove a bus then found a job as a postal employee. They settled in a government housing project for veterans of color after my mother discovered she was pregnant with me. I was born in the spring of 1947 and my brother soon followed in the late summer of 1948. We lived in a small barracks styled house with one bedroom. My brother and I slept in the living room. My mother continued domestic work and discovered she was pregnant again despite the crude birth control of the day, douches and animal skinned condoms. I don't think she was ever fitted for a diaphragm so she used what was available to her, the services of a nurse who performed abortions.

My mother availed herself of the woman's skill two more times because she simply couldn't feed another baby. She said that the nurse was constantly busy because abortion was considered birth control in those days and most of the women she knew had undergone at least one. She never took her decision lightly but to my knowledge didn't dwell on terminating a pregnancy either. Since there was no effective birth control in the early 1950's, there was none of the consternation or religious fervor that permeates the topic today. Women didn't allow men to be involved and the issue was rarely discussed. I knew mother was a lapsed Catholic and once asked her about the church. She simply declared that the Pope wasn't going to feed any of her children or change a shitty diaper and besides, it wasn't any of his business anyway. I was in full agreement. Later, when a childhood friend found herself faced with an unwanted pregnancy, my mother gave her the address of a doctor who could intervene and terminate her pregnancy. When I was a young woman, pre-Roe, several of my friends went to Mexican doctors or found referrals from physicians and friends. Personally, I have never known a woman who ended a pregnancy casually and wasn't emotionally affected but I have also never known a woman who regretted her decision.

F

Failed abortion – with all abortion methods there is a small possibility of the method failing and the pregnancy continuing. Failure rates are given for individual methods. Although available information is not very extensive or accurate it does appear that children born after a pregnancy where there has been a failed medical termination may have higher than average rates of abnormalities.

Fainman, Jack – Winnipeg, Manitoba doctor who was shot on November 11, 1997 by an anti-abortion activist.

Fallopian tubes – tubular structures leading from the uterus to the ovaries (left and right). The fallopian tube is the site of fertilization i.e. it is in the outer third of the tube that the sperm joins with the ovum (egg) to form the zygote that later develops into the embryo and fetus. The fallopian tube is also the most common site of an ectopic pregnancy. Female sterilization is performed by occluding both tubes using clips or rings, or by surgically removing all or part of the tube.

Family planning – see contraception.

Family Planning Associations – non-government not-for-profit organizations in most Australian states that provide information and services in the field of sexual and reproductive health including provision of contraception and advice about pregnancy options including referral for abortion.

FDA – see Food and Drug Administration

Fecundity – the ability to become pregnant within one menstrual cycle.

Federal Abortion Ban – unconstitutional and unenforceable ban on abortions as early as 12 weeks, signed into law by President George W. Bush in 2003. Has been found unconstitutional by six federal courts. Also known as the 'Partial Birth Abortion Ban Act of 2003.' In June 2006 the US Supreme Court announced that it would review the constitutionality of the law. This is considered by many to be an ominous challenge to Roe vs. Wade.

Fellatio – oral stimulation of the penis.

Feminist – activist for women's rights.

Fertile – capable of reproducing

Fertility, in future pregnancies – Strong evidence exists that in countries where induced abortion is legal, a woman who has an uncomplicated abortion performed is not at increased risk of problems with fertility in the future. Where an abortion has been complicated by infection, especially severe pelvic inflammatory disease, it is likely that future fertility may be compromised by the involvement of the fallopian tubes in the infective process. This results in scarring and blockage of the tubes. Exact figures for the incidence of this complication are not readily available.

Fertility Control Clinic – established in East Melbourne, Australia, in 1972 by Dr Bertram Wainer and Jo Wainer following the Wainers' successful attempts to make abortion a public issue and remove police corruption. The clinic offered safe accessible abortion to Victorian women.

Fertilization – the union of a spermatocyte with an ovum.

Fetal – relating to the fetus.

Fetal loss – spontaneous abortion.

Feticide – intentional destruction of the embryo or fetus in the uterus.

Fetus – the developing offspring in the uterus from the seventh week of gestation until birth.

Florida – rated D by **NARAL**. Abortion after 12 weeks is banned and is defined as a felony. Has thus far been found unconstitutional. Only physicians are allowed to perform abortions under Florida law. Florida law allows health care providers or facilities to refuse on religious grounds. to provide information or services related to abortion or contraception. A mandatory counseling law, requiring that the physician tell the woman in person of the nature and risks of 'undergoing or not undergoing' the proposed procedure, the gestational age of the fetus, and the medical risks to both mother and fetus of carrying the pregnancy to term. It also requires that the woman be given state-prepared materials describing the fetus, a list of agencies offering alternatives to abortion and information about medical assistance to carry the pregnancy to term. The enactment of this law is stayed under an injunction; it has been found unconstitutional, but the finding is pending appeal. In Florida, public funding for abortion is prohibited unless the woman's life is endangered. A woman under 18 may not obtain an abortion until 48 hours after notice is given to one parent, either in person or by telephone by the physician. If this is not possible, the procedure must wait until 72 hours after sending notice by certified mail, return receipt requested. A minor woman is not subject to this requirement if she has been married, emancipated by a court or already has a child. There is no provision for waiver in cases of rape or incest unless the woman obtains a court order. Florida imposes a variety of requirements on abortion providers that are not imposed on other health care providers, some of which raise questions of patient privacy. The Florida Constitution protects the right to reproductive choice to a greater extent than the US Constitution. A 2004 amendment to the state constitution removed the right to privacy for minors in respect to abortion.

Folic acid – a B vitamin; deficiency in pregnancy may cause fetal anomalies.

Food and Drug Administration – US federal agency in charge of protecting the public health by assuring the purity and safety of foods, and ensuring that cosmetics and other chemical substances with which people come in contact are safe, effective and honestly labeled. By law, the agency requires prior evidence of safety testing for drugs, food additives, food colorings, cosmetics and pesticides. It also critiques drug tests for efficacy.

Forceps – an instrument resembling tongs or pincers used for grasping, compressing, manipulating, extracting, applying traction, cutting or crushing.

   obstetrical forceps – used to guide the passage of the fetal head through the birth canal and to apply gentle traction to assist the birth.

France – liberal legal grounds for abortion in first ten weeks, but must be requested by the woman through a complex legal process. The result has been no decline in the number of French nationals leaving France to obtain abortions abroad. The incidence of legal abortion in France has not declined since 1983 and is around 21% of all pregnancies. There is a mandatory **'cooling-off' period** of seven days between a woman's presenting for consultation/counseling and the performance of an abortion. Both surgical and medical abortions are available – approximately one third of abortions in France are now medical abortions. **Mifepristone/misoprostol** combinations are widely available and the abortion process in many centers can take place in the woman's home rather than in a hospital or clinic, with access to emergency services if needed.

G

Gerry

I was a rebellious kid, the daughter of a college professor and a permissive mother who had anger management issues. I was the youngest of three sisters and the only one who was never on a scholarly path. I became sexually active at fifteen and it profoundly changed my life. After numerous fights with my parents and sisters, I dropped out of school and left home at sixteen for a life of sex, drugs, and rock n' roll. I supported myself as an under-aged exotic dancer, had numerous sexual encounters and promptly got pregnant. Abortion was legal in the US and as a teen I simply wanted to end my pregnancy and never had any thoughts about having a child; of course, considering the amount of drugs and alcohol I was consuming, there was no way I could have had a normal pregnancy. Still, while I put on a brave front, I had numerous regrets about the abortion but knew it was the best thing I could have done at the time. I was simply too hedonistic to be a decent parent and considering my taste in men, the sperm donor was certainly not daddy material.

I continued pushing the envelope, traveled the US and was able to see Italy and France. Though I had a veneer of polish and certainly was better read then the average stripper, I was still dancing in clubs when I moved to Florida and settled down with a wealthy businessman. I was in my early twenties when I had my second pregnancy, a far different experience from the first. I actually wanted the child though the father did not. It ended in another abortion, this one late term at the end of the second trimester. If I had it to do all over again, I probably would have still terminated my pregnancy but the whole experience left me an emotional mess. I had tremendous regrets but resolved not to get pregnant again. I still romanticize the concept of motherhood especially when I am involved in a relationship but realize that I am simply too self-involved to make a good mother; though my days as a dancer are behind me, I still am a bit a wild child though I have since reconciled with my family and am now the aunt of a little girl whom I adore.

G

Gamete – one of the reproductive cells – an ovum or a spermatocyte.

Gemeprost – drug used to induce abortion usually in the second trimester (16-20+ weeks of pregnancy). Gemeprost is a synthetic prostaglandin that acts to cause a 'mini labour' with the expulsion from the uterus of the fetus, placenta and membranes. Gemeprost was used in early trials of medical abortion in conjunction with mifepristone but **misoprostol** has since been found to be more effective.

Gender – sex i.e. male or female

Gene – a unit carrying the information of heredity located at a fixed position on the chromosome. A gene consists of a segment of DNA containing the code for a specific function or characteristic.

> **X-linked** – carried on the X or female chromosome.

> **Y-linked** – carried on the Y or male chromosome and therefore occurring only in males.

Generative – pertaining to reproduction.

Genetic – determined by genes; hereditary.

Genetics – the study of heredity or in other words, the study of how specific traits are passed from parents to offspring.

Genitalia – the genitals

Genitals – the organs of reproduction.

Genome – the full genetic information in a chromosome.

Genotype – the full set of genes carried by an individual.

Georgia – rated D by **NARAL.** Only physicians are allowed to perform abortions in Georgia. Any person or facility objecting on moral or religious grounds to abortion may refuse to provide abortion information or services. This refusal must be submitted in writing. Similarly, any employee of a state agency that provides contraceptive services may refuse on religious grounds to participate in the same. Georgia also applies regulations to abortion providers that are not applied to other health care providers. For example, all abortions after 13 weeks must be performed in hospitals. Also, abortion facilities must be available at all times for inspection by state officials, with no reference to patient privacy or services. Georgia employs mandatory counseling and waiting periods. Georgia prohibits the use of public funds for abortion unless the woman's life is endangered by a physical cause or the pregnancy is the result of rape or incest. A woman under 18, who has never been married and who is not emancipated, may not obtain an abortion until 24 hours after actual verbal notice to a parent or 72 hours after notification by certified mail, return receipt requested. Notice may not be waived in cases of rape, incest or child abuse. Georgia law requires that any health insurance plan covering prescription drugs also cover contraception.

Germany – abortion is legal, virtually on request to 12 weeks gestation, and up to 22 weeks in cases of fetal abnormality and pregnancy occurring as the result of a crime. Approximately 130,000 abortions are performed annually, almost all surgical. For reasons involving the administration and funding of German health services medical abortion using mifepristone/misoprostol has not become widely used in Germany and many women pay for their own abortions. Counseling by a physician not performing the abortion is mandatory and there is a 3 day **'cooling-off' period**.

Gestation – development of the fetus in the uterus from fertilization until birth.

Gonad – the sexual glands, ovary and testis

Gonadotropin – any hormone that stimulates the ovary or testis.

      human chorionic – a protein hormone produced by the early cells forming the placenta. Secretion of this hormone begins soon after implantation of the fertilized ovum and is the basis of tests for pregnancy.

Gonorrhea – a common sexually transmitted disease, caused by *Neisseria gonorrhoea*. If untreated, it may lead to pelvic infection and infertility.

Gossypol – a substance from cottonseed oil that was viewed with promise as a male contraceptive agent but was found to have too high an incidence of side effects.

Gravid – pregnant.

Gravida – a pregnant woman.

Gravidity – the total number of pregnancies a woman has had.

Griffin, Michael – convicted of murder of Dr. David Gunn, whom he shot in Pensacola, FL in 1993. Sentenced to life imprisonment.

Gunn, David – doctor who performed abortions and who was murdered by Michael Griffin, an anti-abortion protester, in Pensacola, FL in 1993. This was the first murder of a healthcare worker by an anti-abortion protester.

Gut – the intestine.

Gyn-, gyneco-, gyno- – prefixes meaning woman.

Gynecologist – a specialist in disorders of the female reproductive and endocrine organs.

Gynecology – the medical/surgical specialty concerned with disorders of the female reproductive and endocrine organs.

H

Helene

Helene was my cousin. We come from a very traditional family in a small Pacific island nation. Our family was very proud of her when Helene gained her high school diploma but worried about her going away to nursing college in the capital city. It was understood that Helene would return home to make a long-arranged marriage once she completed the course (much as I had when I finished teacher training). In the capital Helene studied hard but she also met Philippe, a boy from a different part of the country, and knowing little of contraception, Helene was soon pregnant. Through friends in the senior year of the course, she was persuaded to see a trained midwife who was willing to help – the woman had performed successful abortions for a number of other students by passing instruments into the womb .Helene's abortion also seemed to be successful – in the beginning. However, two days later she became very ill with fever and although eventually her friends took her to her own teaching hospital, where antibiotics were given, Helene became unconscious and died within hours from the complications of her abortion.

H

Habitus – physical and constitutional characteristics of a person; posture.

Hale, Edwin M – homeopathic physician who published A *Systematic Treatise on Abortion* in 1866. His review of Massachusetts stillbirth statistics from 1840 – 1855 indicated a ratio of one fetal death to every 3 live births. Hale condoned abortion for victims of seduction and wrote that abortion, when skillfully performed, need not be overly dangerous. In his writings for the lay public, however, he allied himself with the AMA anti-abortion stance.

Harris, Elisha M – well-known public health reformer and during the 1860s, Registrar of Vital Statistics of New York City. He was most instrumental in supplying data to Dr. Horatio R. Storer and Franklin Fiske Heard for their compilation of abortion statistics.

Hawaii – rated B+ by **NARAL**. Hawaii permits only physicians to perform abortions. It requires that abortions be performed in hospitals or other specialized facilities. Under Hawaii law, no provider or facility may be required to perform abortions and they are not held liable for failing to provide services or information. Hawaiian law requires any health insurance plan covering prescription drugs to provide equitable coverage for contraception except when such plan is bought by a religious employer for whom such coverage is contrary to their beliefs. Pharmacists are allowed to provide emergency contraception to women without a prescription. Women who are eligible for medical assistance in Hawaii have access to abortion.

Healing – the process of restoring to health.

Heard, Franklin Fiske – lawyer who, together with Dr. Horatio Storer, in 1868, published the most careful and systematic compilation of abortion statistics in America until that time. They reported the ratio of reported early abortions to living births to be 1 to 4.04.

Hemorrhage – profuse bleeding.

    antepartum hemorrhage – occurring at the onset of labor.

    dysfunctional uterine hemorrhage – abnormal uterine bleeding without an identifiable cause.

    fetomaternal hemorrhage – leakage of red blood cells from the fetus to the maternal circulation.

    intraventricular hemorrhage – bleeding into the ventricles of the brain, most commonly in premature babies within 72 hours of birth.

    postpartum hemorrhage – excessive bleeding following vaginal or cesarean delivery.

Hemorrhoids – a swelling of superficial veins around the anus.

Hemostasis – the control of bleeding.

Hepatitis – an inflammation of the liver .Commonly caused by viruses and classified as:

    hepatitis A – transmitted through food or water and does not produce a chronic or carrier state. In pregnancy, only slightly increases the risk of pre-term delivery and is not usually transmitted to the baby. Immunization is available.

    hepatitis B – transmitted by contact with infected blood e.g., by transfusion, contaminated needles, sexually and from mother to baby during birth or breastfeeding. Infection does increase the risk of pre-term delivery and there does exist a chronic and a carrier state. Immunization is available.

hepatitis C – transmitted by contact with infected bodily fluids, contaminated hypodermic needles and contaminated drug paraphernalia. May be sexually transmitted and from mother to baby. A chronic state exists and may lead to liver failure. Common in drug users.

Hill, Paul – a Presbyterian minister and anti-abortion activist, convicted of 1994 murder of Dr. John Britton and women's health clinic volunteer, retired Air Force Lt. Col. James Barrett. Also severely injured in the attack was June Barrett, a retired nurse who, with her husband, was a clinic escort as part of her church ministry. Hill was sentenced to death, resulting in a campaign to commute his sentence to life imprisonment. This campaign was joined by the families of his victims, Amnesty International and many others, on the grounds both that Hill not be granted 'martyrdom' and that killing another person was no way to end the violence. Hill was executed 3 Sept., 2003. He expressed no remorse for his deeds and said that he expected a great reward in Heaven.

History of abortion in the United States – Prior to 1825, the legal attitude toward abortion was that of English common law: quickening or the first sensation of movement in the womb, which occurs late in the fourth month or early in the fifth, was the accepted sign that the fetus had life. Prior to quickening, termination of the pregnancy – often termed 'obstructed menses' or 'blocked menses' – was considered not criminal at all. Home medical manuals of the time gave explicit information on 'relieving obstructed menses' and on things to avoid in suspected pregnancy lest a miscarriage be inadvertently triggered. Medical journals prior to 1840 indicated that abortion was not uncommon and that its primary use was in unmarried women who had 'illicit' intercourse and not as a means of family planning.

The earliest laws relating to the legal status of abortion were enacted between 1821 and 1841. The first of these laws was passed in Connecticut in 1821 and was primarily concerned with attempted murder by poisoning and by extension of the potential for poisoning by the various purgatives and herbal mixtures in vogue as abortifacients. The law did not condemn abortion per se, but declared illegal one method of procuring abortion with an intention of protecting the life and health of the mother. It also held the woman blameless and only referred to the person who caused the poison to be administered. It is important to note that this law reaffirmed the 'quickening doctrine' by stating that a person could be convicted under this law only if the poison was administered to a 'woman quick with child.' In 1830, the law was revised, making abortion by any method after quickening a punishable offense, with punishment of 7 to 10 years imprisonment.

In 1825, Missouri and 1827, Illinois, passed laws very similar to the 1821 Connecticut law, with the difference that neither made explicit reference to the quickening doctrine. These laws made the administration of poison with the intent of causing abortion illegal at any stage of gestation. However, because it was impossible to ascertain pregnancy before quickening it was impossible to prosecute prior to quickening. Missouri proscribed surgical abortion in 1835 and Illinois did so in 1867.

A New York law passed in 1828 addressed abortion. It banned abortion by any means after quickening. An early abortion remained legal, the death of an 'unborn quick child' was second-degree manslaughter and the person who performed the abortion was criminally liable, not the woman herself. In order for the crime to exist, either the woman or the fetus had to die; therefore, an unsuccessful abortion was not considered a crime. An important provision written into this New York law was for therapeutic abortion. It made punishable the willful intent to cause abortion by any means whatever unless the procedure was necessary to save the life of the woman, or if two physicians declared the necessity of abortion for the life of the woman. The notes of the commission undertaking the writing of this law shed light on the intent of these provisions: they were to protect women from incautious medical practitioners whose zeal for operating might be balanced by the consultation of two experienced practitioners. This was in the context of a time when any surgical procedure was very dangerous.

In 1834, Ohio passed a law making attempted abortion a misdemeanor. This made no distinction between stages of gestation. It made the death of the mother or fetus after quickening a felony. Other provisions of this law made it an offense for any physician to prescribe while drunk or to sell secret remedies that endangered life.

In 1835, Indiana added a law similar to Ohio's but Indiana did not make death after quickening a felony. In 1859, Indiana added a proscription against advertising medicine with the intent of procuring abortion.

In 1837, Arkansas made abortion after quickening manslaughter.

In 1839, Iowa passed a poison control measure similar to Connecticut, Missouri and Illinois, but made no further reference to abortion. In the same year, Mississippi made abortion after quickening second-degree manslaughter.

In 1841, Alabama made abortion after quickening a crime.

In 1840, Maine made attempted abortion of any pregnant woman an offense regardless of quickening or particular method used. The law included a therapeutic exception if the mother's life was endangered. While this law eliminated the quickening doctrine, it was difficult to prosecute because of the difficulty of proving intent.

All of the laws passed between 1821 and 1841 punished only the perpetrator of the abortion attempt; none punished the woman herself. The intent of the laws was clearly more to regulate the activities of physicians and apothecaries than to dissuade women from abortion.

In the 1840s, the pattern of abortions in the US began to change. The fact that Americans practiced abortion became an obvious social reality, the incidence of abortion markedly increased, remaining high into the 1880s, and the demographics of abortion changed to a sharp increase in use for family planning purposes by middle and upper-class married American women. In the 1840s, abortion became a free market enterprise, with practitioners advertising their services in the lay press in both urban and rural areas. The abortion business was lucrative and competitive. Competence of the practitioners varied from grossly incompetent to those with good medical training.

In 1845, Massachusetts passed the first law that made attempted abortion at any stage of pregnancy punishable by jail and fines. The law covered any means by which abortion was attempted. Over the following decade, there were thirty-two trials in Massachusetts for attempted abortion, but no convictions. In 1847, the Massachusetts legislature further strengthened the law by outlawing all advertising of abortion or contraceptive services and products.

In 1845, New York State also revised its abortion legislation. This law specifically nullified all preceding state law on the subject. Section one made the death of either the woman or fetus second-degree murder. Section two, which was aimed at commercial abortionists, made any attempt to abort a pregnant woman by any means punishable by a jail term of from three to twelve months. In fact, this provision proved unenforceable in cases of pregnancy prior to quickening because pregnancy could not be proven in those cases. The third provision was unprecedented: the woman herself was liable to punishment for seeking and procuring an abortion or for attempting to perform one on herself. The law retained the therapeutic exception in cases of danger to the life of the mother.

In 1846, Michigan made abortion at any time punishable by jail or fine and abortion after quickening manslaughter. The law provided an exception for the preservation of the life of the mother or when two physicians advised of the necessity of the abortion. In the same year, Vermont passed a law making attempted abortion on a pregnant woman a felony if the woman died as a result.

In 1848, Virginia passed a law stating that the death of a pre-quickened fetus was punishable by up to twelve months in jail and that of a quickened fetus by up to five years imprisonment. The law was virtually unenforceable because of the difficulty of proving the crime. In 1849, Wisconsin made abortion a crime only when performed on a woman pregnant with a 'quick child' and California passed a law requiring that the woman be proven pregnant. In 1858, Wisconsin added a clause making any woman who attempted to procure or self-induce an abortion culpable under law.

Also in1849, New Hampshire passed its first anti-abortion law. The law that passed provided that attempted abortion at any stage of pregnancy was punishable by up to one year in jail or a $1000 fine, abortion after quickening with imprisonment for one to ten years, plus the fine, and made the abortionist guilty of second-degree manslaughter if the woman should die. The law also became the second in US history to make the woman herself culpable and subject to criminal punishment.

New Jersey law, passed in 1849, preserved the woman's immunity against prosecution and made her welfare paramount. The law made all attempts at abortion illegal, as well as offering advice or instructions on how to abort a fetus was also illegal and the law provided harsher punishment should the woman die. In a test of the law before the New Jersey Supreme Court in 1857, the finding was that the intent of the law was to protect the life and health of the mother and that the life of the fetus was immaterial in the intent of the law. The woman was regarded as the victim of the crime.

Minnesota Territory, in 1851, and Oregon Territory, in 1854, outlawed abortion after quickening and before quickening if the woman was injured. Kansas Territory in 1855 made attempted abortion at any time a misdemeanor, but required proof of pregnancy and intent. Washington Territory in 1854 made it an offense to abort any pregnant woman or any woman presumed to be pregnant.

In 1854, Texas made abortion after quickening a crime punishable by up to ten years in prison. In 1856, this prison term was reduced to between two and five years if the woman had consented. This revision also added a definition of abortion-related deaths as murder, made anyone supplying abortifacients an accomplice to the crime, and added the therapeutic exception for the life and health of the woman. In 1858, they further clarified that the attempt itself, whether successful or not, was criminal.

Louisiana, in 1856, made procuring an abortion or 'premature delivery' of any pregnant woman a felony punishable by up to ten years imprisonment.

Horatio Robinson Storer, a young obstetrician/gynecologist, in 1857 used the newly-formed American Medical Association (1847) as a launching pad for a nation-wide campaign for suppression of the 'abominable, unnatural and common crime' of abortion. At the AMA's 1859 national convention, a resolution was adopted citing ignorance on the part of the general population in regard to the significance of quickening, supposed indifference by some members of the profession to fetal life, and the 'grave defects' of the laws. In remedy, the AMA resolved to protest the quickening doctrine, urge revision of the various state and territorial abortion laws, and enjoined the various state medical societies to join in the efforts of the AMA. The AMA also voted against a recommendation in 1868 by their ethics committee that consultation be permitted between its members and female physicians and against allowing membership or affiliation with schools that allowed women to study medicine.

Between 1860 and 1880, many consumer health manuals appeared in press. These had the intent of educating the public to the dangers of abortion and toward an anti-abortion moral code. Edwin M. Hale, professor at Hahnemann College, a homeopathic medical school, and a leading homeopath opposed abortion in principle but considered abortion safe and sometimes necessary. In 1866, he published a textbook on abortion that claimed that abortion performed by skillful operators was not unduly risky and that in no case should the life and/or health of the mother be sacrificed to save a fetus before viability of the fetus. Protestant clergy did not become conspicuously and unanimously involved in the campaign for abortion law reform. Catholic clergy made their alignment with the AMA known, but were not a major force in the campaign.

In 1873, Congress passed the Comstock Act, an act for the 'suppression of trade in and circulation of obscene literature and articles of immoral use' or, in other words, an anti-obscenity law. This law, which was intended to deter trade in pornography, was also extended to abortion and contraceptive related advertising and the publishing of books, tracts and articles related to the same. Anthony Comstock, head of the New York Society for the Suppression of Vice, was made an agent of the federal government and in effect, became the anti-obscenity czar of the era. He was empowered to enforce the law and for the remainder of the 1870s aggressively pursued and prosecuted abortionists under this law. Among others caught in his net was Madame Restell who committed suicide prior to her trial in 1878.

A significant change in law occurred in 1860, when Connecticut passed new anti-abortion legislation. This law had four sections: 1) affirmed Connecticut's opposition to abortion, making no mention of quickening, and making abortion a felony, punishable by a fine of up to $1000 and imprisonment of up to five years; 2) accomplices to the act were considered felons, as well; 3) the woman herself was guilty of a felony for soliciting an abortion, permitting one to be performed on her or for attempting to abort herself; 4) advertising or disseminating materials relating to abortion was illegal and subject to fines of up to $500.

Pennsylvania, in 1860, revised their anti-abortion statute to make any attempted abortion illegal, regardless of proof of pregnancy.

Oregon, in 1864, passed the only abortion legislation acted upon during the Civil War. This removed the quickening doctrine from their previous legislation and made any purposeful destruction of any 'child' in utero manslaughter, regardless of whether the woman came to any harm.

After the Civil War, the coupling of increased influence of the 'regular' physicians, due to better training and access to improved medical knowledge, with a political climate favorable to the influence of these physicians and the anti-abortion campaign of their organization, the AMA, many states strengthened their abortion laws. Alabama increased the penalties for performing an abortion. Florida addressed abortion-related death after quickening and made any attempted abortion, regardless of gestational age or harm to the woman, punishable by fine and imprisonment. Louisiana made surgical abortion illegal in addition to its previous proscription on abortifacient drugs. Illinois in 1867, increased the penalties for performing an abortion and defined the crime as murder if the woman died. This law exempted only those abortions performed for bona fide medical or surgical reasons. Further, in 1871, Illinois passed a bill prohibiting sales and advertisement of abortifacient agents. In Ohio, a special report by the legislators indicated concern about the failure of the American family, in that abortion was seen as being used to limit family size and was common and publicly tolerated. The resulting law passed by the legislature made illegal abortion at any gestational stage, deleting the quickening doctrine. They also passed legislation intended to prevent the advertising and sale of any medicines or substances for the purpose of inducing abortion. Under the same influences, Vermont in 1867, made it illegal for any person to attempt abortion not only on any pregnant woman, but also on any woman believed to be pregnant. The woman herself was specifically held immune to penalty. The sale and advertising of abortifacients or dissemination of information was also made illegal and punishable by fines and imprisonment.

In 1867, Colorado Territory added a therapeutic exception that went beyond the common exemption for the life of the mother. This law also allowed abortion upon the advice of a physician or surgeon not only to save the life of the woman, but also to 'prevent serious and permanent bodily injury to her.'

Maryland, in 1867, passed a law providing for the licensure of doctors to "protect the public against medical imposters" and provided harsh penalties for performing an abortion and outlawed all advertising or purveyance of abortifacients and abortion services. Under the law, informers were to be rewarded. In 1868, this law was watered down by adding the word "knowingly" before many of the proscriptions and by specifically allowing medical practitioners to 'supervise and manage' any abortion that has occurred spontaneously from any cause. . . allowing doctors to help women who may have tried to self-abort or having seen an unskilled abortionist and who then presented to the doctor. It also allowed abortion on the consultation of one or more "respectable physicians." It also removed the rewards for informers.

New York, in 1868, passed a law forbidding the publication of materials relating to abortion advertising, information and other practices deemed obscene. In 1869, the legislature revised its abortion law to make abortion at any gestational stage second-degree manslaughter, made attempted abortion of any woman, pregnant or not, a misdemeanor and made all parties to an abortion competent witnesses to the abortion and granted said witnesses immunity against prosecution. In 1872, this was further amended to make the abortion-related death of the woman or the fetus a felony, made any woman who submitted to an abortion or aborted herself guilty of a felony, made illegal attempts at abortion, successful or not, at any stage of gestation, and forbade the advertising, manufacture or sale of any abortifacient materials. In 1875, a further addition to the law was the admissibility as evidence of the dying declarations of a woman whose death was abortion related.

Similar tightening of anti-abortion laws occurred in Massachusetts, Nevada and Wyoming in 1869. Michigan in 1871 passed a law outlawing the publication and sale of any literature relating to the cures for 'female complaints or private diseases' and the recipes or prescription for any substance designed to produce abortion or miscarriage, except "upon the written order of any physician." Pennsylvania and Kansas passed similar laws in 1870 and 1874, respectively.

In 1872, a woman who voluntarily submitted to abortion or who tried to abort herself became guilty of a crime for the first time under California law. In the same year, New Jersey made feticide a crime in and of itself. In 1873, Minnesota, Virginia and Nebraska changed their official attitudes of ambiguity to official aggressive opposition to abortion. In 1875, Arkansas added to its proscription against abortion of a 'quick child' equal proscription against abortion of any fetus before quickening. It also added similar provisions against advertising and selling of abortion information and abortifacient materials to that of other states. In 1876, Georgia made abortion an assault with intent to murder and attempted abortion a misdemeanor.

Prior to 1880, despite anti-abortion laws being in place, local and state courts tended to demand a very high burden of proof in abortion cases and seldom found the accused guilty. This began to change around 1880 and more and more decisions were made against the accused and the burden of proving that an abortion was performed to save the woman's life was placed upon the person accused of performing the abortion. The quickening doctrine became out-of-date, as did proof that the woman was pregnant. Documents of the time, indicate that between 1880 and 1900, abortion rates were declining, that it was resorted to by fewer married women as a method of limiting their families and that in this time period, it was resorted to more frequently by unmarried and lower-class women, a distinct change in demographics from earlier.

There was little substantive change in abortion laws until the 1973 Roe vs. Wade decision of the United States Supreme Court. This decision found the Texas anti-abortion law unconstitutional and by extension all similar states' laws. The Supreme Court found that during the first trimester of pregnancy, a woman's right to privacy takes precedence. During the second trimester, the right of the state to regulate and protect female health prevailed: the state could not deny a woman an abortion but could regulate the standards of the medical procedures of abortion. During the third trimester, the Court found that the state might proscribe abortion except when necessary to preserve the life or health of the mother. See further explication under Roe vs. Wade.

For current individual state laws, see the alphabetical listings for the individual states, which for ease of reading have not been included in bold type for this history.

Hodgson, Jane – prominent obstetrician/gynecologist in St. Paul, MN who, in 1971, became the only physician in US history to be convicted of performing an abortion in a hospital. Hodgson performed this procedure as a challenge to the Minnesota law on abortion.

Horsley, Neal – posts a website known to anti-abortion activists as the "Nuremburg files." This site lists names and addresses of doctors and abortion clinic personnel, as well as judges and politicians who "pass or uphold laws authorizing child-killing." President George W. Bush was added to the list in Aug., 2001, after announcing limited support of stem-cell research. The names of people killed are crossed out and people who have been injured are grayed out.

Hydatidiform mole – uncommon condition occurring in pregnancy in which the fetus fails to develop but the placenta develops into a rapidly expanding but benign tumor, the 'mole'. Very rarely a fetus may also be present with the mole. Hydatidiform mole is a cause of bleeding in early pregnancy. The uterus requires emptying by suction curettage and the woman requires close follow-up as rarely hydatidiform mole progresses to become malignant.

I

Isabella

My story could wear many names and many faces. I was in my late teens and giddily in love with Herman. He was well built, with bronzed skin and shining dark hair and flashing white teeth and his touch made me feel a little bit dizzy with longing. It started with brief meetings after work, to sit over a soda while he smoked a cigarette, but then it progressed to taking long walks and going to the movies. Within three months, we had become lovers and I was ecstatically happy. I felt as though no harm could touch me because this good man loved me.

After six months, I noticed that my breasts were very tender, more than usual before my period. The period came and went, but the tenderness persisted and I began to feel a little nauseated when I was cooking and when I was hungry. The second month, I had no period. Alarmed, I went to my mother, who bought a home pregnancy test and helped me to do it. It was positive. "You've got to tell him right away, girl."

Feeling very fragile and tentative, I offered my news to Herman as though I were handing him a precious gift. Herman turned very pale and then asked how could this be? He had always used protection. "Have you been going with somebody else, too? Must be, 'cause I ain't made any kid."

I was shaking as I assured Herman that I had been faithful and that one of the rubbers must have leaked or something... "But we love each other, so it'll be OK, won't it?"

"Sure, it'll be OK. You can get rid of it. I'll give you the money and I'll even go with you to the clinic. We don't need no kid cluttering up our lives right now. You just make the appointment and I'll be there with you."

I made the appointment, which was scheduled for the next week. The night before, I talked with my mother about it and realized that I was feeling very sad and angry and somehow abused. I didn't think that a pregnancy arising from the love I felt for Herman should be so easily dismissed. My mother understood. "If you want to have this baby and raise it, you won't be the first woman to raise her child without its daddy – are you sure he wouldn't agree to raising it? Anyway, you have me and I'll help you as much as I can."

When I told Herman that I wanted to have the baby, he went ballistic. "You're like all women. You just want to put shackles on a man and tie him to a bunch of kids and a go-nowhere job. Not me. I'm getting out of this place and going to the city and make me a bunch of money before I settle down. You might have been part of it, but now you go and ruin it."

Obviously, I was devastated. I called in sick to my job for a couple of days, stayed in bed, and cried. Late the second afternoon, I got up, made a meal for myself and my mother and realized that I felt very calm and resolved. While we ate, I told my mother that I planned to cancel the clinic appointment and make one with our family doctor to begin prenatal care. "Whatever Herman felt, I conceived this baby in love, and I'm not going to get rid of it. Maybe it would be different if I was all alone, but I have you. We're strong women, Momma."

Momma was a strong support in the months that followed; she helped me sign up for Medicaid since I was not covered by any health insurance and together we prepared to make a home for a child. The pregnancy was complicated by gestational diabetes, and I had to quit work in my seventh month, but Momma took care of me and went to her own job, too. Momma was there at the delivery of Emelia, another link in the chain of strong women.

Today, I'm married to Tom. Tom is about six years older than I am and has a little boy from a previous marriage. We met at work, when Tom was transferred to be the manager of the store where I clerked. The marriage is five years old now and it is a good marriage. Momma has retired from her job and takes care of Emelia and Jake, Tom's son (now mine, too) while we work.

I

Iatrogenic – caused by medical diagnosis or treatment.

Ibuprofen – a non-aspirin, nonsteroidal anti-inflammatory drug, used to treat pain and as an anti-prostaglandin.

Idaho – rated F by **NARAL**. Idaho has an unconstitutional and unenforceable ban on abortion as early as twelve weeks; it also has added an intent to restrict the right to choice in its state code. Idaho mandates counseling by the physician, including a description of the intended procedure, an explanation of any risks or adverse effects associated with the procedure, including future reproductive sequelae, and the comparable risks associated with each alternative to abortion, including childbirth and adoption. It further requires the provision of state-prepared materials detailing the developmental stages of the fetus, services available to the woman during and after pregnancy and childbirth, including adoption services, descriptions of the various abortion procedures and the risks attendant upon them; a woman may not have an abortion until 24 hours after receiving these materials. Idaho permits only physicians to perform legal abortions and has an unconstitutional and unenforceable law that subjects abortion providers to restrictions not placed on other medical providers. Idaho law provides for any health care worker or hospital or physician's employee to refuse to participate in abortion related services. The refusal must be tendered in writing. Similarly, it provides for the same people to refuse to participate in sterilization procedures. Under Idaho law, managed care insurance plans, individual health insurance policies and disability policies must exclude coverage for abortion unless it is necessary to preserve the woman's life. Coverage may be obtained by payment of an additional premium from those carriers that offer it. Idaho provides that no abortion may be performed after viability unless two physicians certify that this is necessary to preserve the woman's life or that the fetus would not survive if born. It defines viable as 'potentially able to live outside the mother's womb, albeit with artificial aid'. It also requires that the physician choose the technique of abortion most apt to preserve the life of the fetus. The lack of a health exception has been deemed unconstitutional by the Idaho Attorney General. Public funds may not be used for abortion in Idaho unless the abortion is necessary to preserve the life of the woman or the pregnancy is the result of rape or incest that has been duly reported. Minor women under 18 may not receive an abortion unless they have written consent from one parent or has obtained a judicial waiver of this provision. This provision may be waived if the physician certifies that a medical emergency exists. This law is unenforceable because the health exception has been deemed inadequate.

Illegal abortion – In a large number of countries – principally in Africa, South America and South East Asia – abortion is illegal, the only exception being to save the mother's life. Countries where abortion is illegal provide most of the annual 70,000+ maternal deaths from the complications of abortion, strong evidence that women will still seek abortions even when these are outside the law. Abortion-related deaths are a major component of maternal mortality in developing countries. Examples of countries where abortion is illegal include Argentina and Cameroon. Argentina allows legal abortion only if the mother's life and/or health are in extreme danger. However, Argentina has one of the highest abortion ratios in the world, with one abortion for every two live births and abortion is the most important cause of death in Argentina in women over 20 years old. In Cameroon abortion is legal only to save the mother's life or for pregnancy resulting from rape, but almost one-third of emergency admissions at the main maternity hospital are due to unsafe illegal abortions. This is estimated to account for between 30 and 40% of maternal deaths. In some countries notably Brazil and Uruguay illegal surgical abortion has been replaced by illegal use of **misoprostol** to bring about medical abortion. Although misoprostol abortion is safest performed under medical supervision, unsupervised misoprostol use is much safer than surgical abortion performed illegally by untrained operators. Consequently death rates from abortion in these countries have been falling.

Illinois – rated C by **NARAL**. Illinois has a ban on abortions after 12 weeks. It has been ruled unconstitutional because it has no exception for a woman's health and because it unduly burdens the right of a woman to choose abortion. Performance of abortion is restricted to physicians. Certain employees or organizations receiving state funds are prohibited from counseling or referring women for abortion. Similarly, insurance funds for state employees may not cover abortion services unless the woman's life is endangered. Illinois has a requirement that the husband of any married woman be notified before she can obtain an abortion; this has been found unconstitutional. Illinois has added anti-choice language to its state code. This language expresses the intent of Illinois to return to a pre-Roe stance of allowing abortion only when the woman's life is endangered if and when Roe should ever be reversed. Any health care provider or facility may refuse in writing to participate in abortion or other health care service on the grounds of conscience. Illinois has a parental notification law for minor (under 18) women but this law has been held unenforceable by a federal court. Illinois imposes a variety of special regulations on abortion providers. Illinois law ensures that all victims of sexual assault have access to emergency contraception. Illinois law also guarantees that a woman can fill her birth control prescriptions. It also requires that all insurance plans covering prescription drugs also cover contraception. Low-income women have access to abortion under the state medical assistance. The Illinois Constitution protects the right to reproductive choice.

Implantation – attachment of the fertilized ovum to the inner wall of the uterus. This begins 5-7 days after fertilization.

Impotence – inability to achieve or maintain an erection of the penis.

Impregnate – to make pregnant.

Incest – sexual activity, including intercourse, between closely related individuals.

Incomplete abortion – an abortion with retained products of conception. This situation is not uncommon with spontaneous abortion (miscarriage.) Only part of the pregnancy (i.e. fetus if one has developed, placenta and membranes) is passed through the vagina. Some tissue remains inside the uterus and while this is the case some bleeding and cramps may continue. If pain and bleeding are not severe it may be possible to wait for the tissue remaining (usually referred to as the products of conception) to be passed naturally. This is likely to take the form of bleeding which may be moderate to heavy but not necessarily so. Alternatively the retained products can be removed surgically with a **D&C.** This is usually done if there is heavy or persistent bleeding or pain and certainly if fever or other sign suggest the possibility of developing infection. Where incomplete abortion follows induced abortion (medical or surgical) again products of conception may pass spontaneously or may be removed surgically depending on the degree of bleeding and pain present.

Incontinence – inability to control the passage of urine or feces.

Indiana – rated F by **NARAL**. The Indiana Constitution protects the right to reproductive choice as a fundamental right. Indiana has a ban on abortion after 12 weeks, but this was held unconstitutional because it did not provide for the health of the woman and was written so broadly that it bans more than one procedure and limits a woman's right to choose. Indiana allows abortion only by physicians and has targeted regulations applied only to abortion providers. Women seeking abortion have to undergo mandated counseling and a mandatory delay. State employees or organizations receiving state funds are prohibited from advocating or promoting abortion, including making reference to it. Individuals or organizations may refuse on religious or moral grounds to provide abortion information, referral or services. Public funding for abortion is prohibited except in those cases in which the woman's life is in danger, she is at risk of 'irreversible impairment of a major bodily function' or the pregnancy is the result of rape or incest. An unemancipated woman under age 18 may not obtain an abortion except with the consent of one parent. There are no exceptions to this except by court order.

Inevitable abortion – This is a form of spontaneous abortion (miscarriage). Pain and bleeding occurs naturally and the cervix dilates (opens) but products of conception have not yet been passed. There is no way of preventing miscarriage from occurring, i.e. the abortion process in inevitable

Infant – person from birth until the age of one year.

> **live-born infant** – an infant who demonstrates evidence of life after being born from mother. This evidence may be a heart beat, pulsation of the umbilical cord, spontaneous respiration, or movement.

> **stillborn infant**– an infant who shows no sign of life at birth.

Infanticide – the intentional killing of an infant.

Infection – Infection of products of conception can occur with both spontaneous and induced abortion, and the infection can spread to the tissues of the mother. Following induced abortion in a clinic or hospital setting, up to one in 10 women experience some degree of infection of the genital tract (vagina, cervix, uterus and fallopian tubes.) This is due to the introduction of organisms ('germs' -usually bacteria) on hands or instruments during the procedure or to the migration of such bacteria from the woman's bowel or skin up into the vagina and hence to the uterus. Another possibility is that the woman already has a mild and symptomless infection such as *Chlamydia* or other sexually-transmitted infection which spreads as a result of the abortion process. The infection may be mild with some vaginal discharge or severe with the development of salpingitis or pelvic inflammatory disease (PID).

The risk of infection is reduced when women are given prophylactic antibiotics before the abortion is performed, or have swabs taken prior to induced abortion and have diagnosed infections treated. Common organisms causing infection that may be diagnosed from swabs prior to induced abortion are *Chlamydia* and the gonococcus, which causes the disease gonorrhea. Antibiotic treatment may be continued following an induced abortion.

Infection can also occur in association with spontaneous abortion, when exactly the same types of organisms may be responsible. Antibiotics should be given and if some tissue remains within the uterus (i.e. there is incomplete abortion) then D&C may be needed to remove this.

Informed consent – see consent.

International Federation of Gynecology and Obstetrics – International organisation of all national colleges of obstetrics and gynecology. Takes the position that preventing unwanted pregnancies and addressing unsafe abortion is an important part of all national safe motherhood programs. Notes that while most national programs focus on wanted pregnancies and childbirth, approximately one third of the estimated 200 million pregnancies worldwide each year are unwanted. Maternal deaths from unsafe abortion account for at least 13% of maternal mortality worldwide. In some countries, unsafe abortion is the most common cause of maternal mortality. In US, mortality rate associated with legal abortion is 0.7 per 100,000.

Intra-vaginally – the administration of medication e.g. misoprostol by placing tablets or pessaries high in the vagina. may be done by physicians, nurses or women themselves.

Iowa – rated C by NARAL. Iowa has a ban on abortion after 12 weeks. This has been held unconstitutional because it imposes an undue burden on women seeking abortions. In Iowa, abortion may be performed only by physicians. No state medical assistance funds or funds appropriated to the State University of Iowa hospitals or clinics may be used to terminate pregnancy unless continuation of the pregnancy endangers the life of the woman, the fetus is deformed or has a congenital illness, or the pregnancy is the result of rape reported within 45 days of occurrence or incest reported within 150 days of occurrence. Any individual or institution not controlled, maintained or supported by public agency may refuse to participate in abortion on moral or religious grounds. A woman under 18 who has never been married may not obtain an abortion until at least 48 hours after one parent is notified in writing. This may be waived if the young woman declares that she is a victim of rape, incest or child abuse and these have been reported. Iowa requires that insurance plans that cover prescription drugs give equitable coverage to contraception.

IPPF – International Planned Parenthood Federation – see Planned Parenthood

Ireland – Abortion is not legal in Ireland; the only exception is to save the life of the woman. In 1983 a referendum resulted in an amendment to the Constitution saying that: 'The State acknowledges the right to life of the unborn and, with due regard to the equal right to life of the mother, guarantees in its laws to respect, and as far as practicable, by its laws to defend and vindicate that right.'

A ruling banning information and counseling on abortion was made in 1985. Ensuing legal battles reached the European Court where it was decided that information and travel to obtain abortion should be allowed by all member states including Ireland. A right to travel abroad for an abortion was established in 1992 and it is widely recognized that every year an estimated 60,000 Irish women travel to the United Kingdom and elsewhere for abortions.

A recent survey carried out by Lansdowne Market Research in Ireland, on behalf of the Abortion Reform lobby group, indicated that 79 per cent of people favored women having limited access to abortion. This survey also found that nearly half of those questioned (47 per cent) supported abortion in cases of rape or incest, and 52 per cent supported abortion when there was a physical threat to the mother's life.

Ireland, Northern – abortion is legal in Northern Ireland as elsewhere in the United Kingdom. However, abortion both surgical and medical is difficult to access. fpaNI (family planning association Northern Ireland) has recently won the right to a judicial review to clarify the circumstances in which abortion may be provided in Northern Ireland.

Islam – attitudes to abortion. The Koran does not specifically address abortion, but it does encourage marital sexual relations and the procreation of children. Islam does not condone abortion except when continuing the pregnancy endangers the life or health of the woman, when abortion is permitted up to 120 days of pregnancy in some Muslim countries. The position of Islam is that a woman does not have ownership of her body, to do as she will with it. Her body is entrusted to her as a sacred gift by Allah and she is obligated to treat it in a pure and holy manner. Islam does allow contraception. Sex before marriage or extra-marital sex is expressly forbidden but sex within marriage is regarded as a benediction on both partners.

Italy – abortion has been legal in Italy since 1978. A referendum in 1981 to try to repeal this law was defeated with only 32% votes in favor of repeal. Around 19% of pregnancies in Italy end in induced abortion; the highest proportion of abortions is in the Pope's own diocese of Rome. Most abortions are surgical – mifepristone/misoprostol abortion has only limited availability at the time of writing and there have been major demonstrations in Italian cities in opposition to the Catholic Church's attempts to have mifepristone banned in Italy.

J

Jackie

I was 40 years old when I had an abortion, so that's three years ago now. I was married to Richard; we'd been married sixteen years by then and had three kids. The youngest, Katie, is 13 now. I was in and out of hospital when I was pregnant with her, because I was hemorrhaging, and so for a lot of that time we didn't have sex. While I was still in hospital getting over the birth I found that Richard had been seeing my so-called 'best friend.' We had a huge row and for a while he moved out but it was really hard with the baby and in the end I took him back. But things were never right with us after that, I could never make love with him without thinking of him being with her.

I'm just trying to explain I guess how I ended up having an affair myself. When Katie went to elementary school, I got a job, just in sales, nothing much but something of my own, and I met him at work. I worked flexi shifts and he would hire a motel room and I would meet him there, Richard didn't know exactly what my hours were and he didn't notice. It sounds sleazy now I know but at the time, well, it seemed exciting. I knew there was no future in it for us. I got condoms but he didn't like them. Richard had a vasectomy after Katie was born but I still had an old diaphragm and I used that. No surprise that about two months later I realized I was pregnant and none I guess that Mr. Romance scooted – just disappeared from work and was never seen again. I had no choice. I had to pawn my mother's engagement ring to get the money because Richard checks all our bank accounts.

I made the decision straight away and because I was just six weeks pregnant I was able to take the mifeprex. I didn't need the second drug because I started to bleed the same day. I told Richard I had a heavy period and that it was normal in women my age, he knows nothing about women's problems anyway. I just took some pain killer and it went all right. I felt terrible about doing it but I knew there was no other choice. I bled for about two weeks after that but not heavily. Then about six months later Richard left me anyway, for a woman he'd met at work. So the world goes…

Katie's my only girl. She's too young yet but when she's older I'll make sure she is really well informed about contraception. I wouldn't want her to go through what I did. But I was glad that I could get the pills legally when I needed them and that it was safe.

J

Jane – an organization formed in 1969 by the Abortion Counseling Service of Women's Liberation. The purpose of the organization was to help women procure safe illegal abortions. All members were known by the pseudonym of "Jane." After realizing that the principal abortionist to whom they were referring women was not a physician, the Janes learned to perform abortions themselves and were soon performing all procedures themselves. See **Heather Booth**

Judaism – the position on abortion taken at the Biennial Convention of the United Synagogue of Conservative Judaism is that Judaism is in support of the availability of legal abortion; that personhood does not begin at conception; that in cases where the life or health of the mother are endangered, abortion is mandated by the Jewish faith; abortion is not condoned for contraceptive purposes; and that to deny a Jewish woman the right to a safe legal abortion when consistent with Jewish tradition, is to deny her religious rights. In Talmudic law, a fetus is deemed part of its mother and a fetus has no independent rights under Talmudic law. Feticide is not considered murder because the fetus is not considered fully human until the moment of birth. Judaism considers the question of ensoulment but dismisses it as irrelevant to abortion because it is irresoluble.

K

Karen

I'm 36. I've lived with my partner Terry for ten years and we have one son, Ben, he's five now. Ben is fantastic, I gave up work when he was born and I just adore him. When he was nearly three we decided to try for another baby, a girl we hoped but it wouldn't have mattered. I fell pregnant straight away.

At my first antenatal clinic visit the doctor asked if I wanted the tests for Down syndrome. It involved an ultrasound and a blood test. He told me the chances of having a baby like that at age 34 were very low but there was no risk to me or the baby from the test. So I said yes. I had the tests about a week later. I didn't hear anything so I thought it must all be okay. Then when I was 13 weeks I got a call from the clinic saying come along urgently. The tests had shown a high risk of Down syndrome but someone had messed up and not looked at the results for about a week. Terry came with me and we were petrified.

The doctor we saw though was really good. He took a lot of time to explain that I could have another test that would definitely tell us if the baby was Down syndrome. Chorionic villous sampling. I had to have a needle through my vagina. They watched the baby on the ultrasound and that was the worst bit, being able to see the baby's arms and legs moving around. Somehow I knew even then what the result would be – and I was right, the tests came back as abnormal. We had already talked it through ourselves and with our priest and knew that we could not cope with a child like that and that it was not in Ben's best interests. We had to make a decision quickly if I wanted a surgical abortion. I had it done with a general anesthetic in a hospital because it was for a medical reason.

I cried non-stop for days. I kept thinking about the baby on the ultrasound and how I wished he or she had been normal and a little brother or sister for Ben. After that I decided I couldn't cope with the anxiety of another pregnancy and I had an IUD put in. I don't think we'd ever try for another child especially as I'm getting older. We're lucky to have Ben.

Yes I did have regrets, a lot of them, about it. As well as Father Paul, I talked to the hospital chaplain and he helped me a lot. I know though now that I did the right thing for all of us, I just wish that the whole thing had never happened.

K

Kansas – rated D- by **NARAL**. Kansas prohibits state employees or organizations receiving state funds from counseling or referring women for abortion. It also prohibits the use of any state-owned medical facilities unless the life or health of the woman is seriously endangered. Under Kansas law, no person associated with healthcare may be required to participate in abortion or sterilization procedures. No woman may have an abortion until 24 hours after receiving in writing from a physician a description of the intended abortion procedure, the name of the physician who will do the procedure, the possible risks and adverse sequelae of the abortion procedure, the gestational age of her fetus and a description of the fetus at this stage, the medical risks of carrying the pregnancy to term and a statement of Kansas' post-viability abortion law. She must also receive state-prepared materials. The post-viability restriction states that no abortion may be performed after viability unless two physicians certify that the abortion is necessary to preserve the woman's life or health. Public funding for abortion is prohibited in Kansas unless the abortion is necessary to preserve the life of the mother or the pregnancy is the result of rape or incest. An unmarried minor woman under the age of 18 may not obtain an abortion until one parent is given notice. This requirement may be waived if the woman declares that the pregnancy is the result of incest with her parent or legal guardian or by judicial waiver or in the case of a medical emergency. She must also receive the mandated counseling while accompanied by a parent or responsible adult over age 21. Kansas law does protect people entering a healthcare facility from obstruction or violence.

Kentucky – rated F by **NARAL**. Kentucky has an unconstitutional and unenforceable ban on abortion as early as 12 weeks. The state code also includes and intent to eliminate reproductive choice. Kentucky law prohibits state employees or organizations receiving state funds from counseling or referring women for abortion. It also prohibits the use of any public facility for abortion. Kentucky has an unconstitutional and unenforceable requirement that the husband of a married woman must be notified before she can obtain an abortion. By law, the emergency services provided to victims of rape or sexual assault must not include abortion counseling or referral. All health insurance contracts in the state must exclude coverage for abortion except when necessary to preserve the woman's life. Coverage may be provided by a rider and additional premium. No state funds may be used to cover abortion services for state employees or their dependents. Only physicians may perform legal abortions in Kentucky and these physicians are subject to a variety of requirements and restrictions not imposed on other physicians. No healthcare personnel or facility may be required to perform abortion services if they are opposed in religious, moral or professional grounds. No abortion may be performed after viability unless it is necessary to preserve the woman's life. No public funding may be used to fund an abortion unless it is necessary to preserve the life of the woman or the pregnancy is the result of incest or rape. In Kentucky, an unmarried woman under the age of 18 may not have an abortion unless she has the written consent of one parent. This requirement may be waived only if the physician certifies that there is a medical emergency requiring the abortion or if the minor obtains a court waiver.

Knight, Peter James – abortion opponent who shot and killed an unarmed security guard, Steven Rogers, outside a Melbourne, Australia, abortion clinic in July 2001. Currently serving a sentence of 23 years for murder.

Kopp, James – murdered Dr. Barnett Slepian in Amherst, NY in Oct. 1998. Kopp shot Dr. Slepian through a kitchen window using a high power assault rifle. The murder was witnessed by Dr. Slepian's wife and children. Kopp confessed to the murder and used as his defense the theory of justifiable homicide because it 'prevented a greater crime.' This thinking was explicated in the 1994 book by Army of God leader Michael Bray. Kopp was also a suspect in four non-fatal shootings of abortion providers in Canada and Rochester, NY. Kopp was found guilty and sentenced to prison for 25 years to life. He had fled to France prior to trial and was extradited back to the US on the provision that he would not face the death penalty.

L

Laura

Jake and I were sweethearts from first grade. We did everything together all through school. Even our parents were best friends. Of course, it was just natural that we would get engaged when we turned eighteen and finished high school. We wanted to get married right away and go away to college together, but my dad said we should try at least a year at different colleges and try out growing a little on our own, away from each other. Then, he said, we could get married the next summer. Jake's parents agreed, so what choice did we have?

Jake and I agreed that we would not sit around and mope at our colleges. We said we'd have fun with groups and go to all the fun activities and then we could share the news with each other. We did this and we talked on the phone every day, until one day Jake didn't call and I couldn't reach him. Same thing the next day. I was steamed! Maybe he was out with some other girl. So I went to the first party I heard about that night and danced and laughed and drank too much. Some parts of the night are a little fuzzy and I don't remember having sex, but I guess I did. When I got up the next day, I called Jake again and when there was no answer, I called his folks. He was in the hospital; two days ago, he had a bad pain in his belly and it turned out to be his appendix. They thought my parents called me with the news and my parents thought Jake's parents had. What a comedy of errors. I got a friend to drive me to the hospital where Jake was and I stayed all that day. I didn't even think to tell him about the party because by then it didn't seem important.

Six weeks later, I found out how important it was. I thought I must have the flu or something because for days I couldn't keep anything down and I was so tired I could barely stay awake in my classes. Finally, I went to the infirmary. The nurse asked a lot of questions, including when my last period was. It had been two months, but I didn't think anything of that because I often skipped and I hadn't had sex since summer (I thought), but she insisted on doing a pregnancy test. When she told me it was positive, I fainted dead away! She was so good to me and gradually we pieced it together and figured that somebody must have slipped me something at that party. Whatever happened, the reality was that I was pregnant.

Now, I was brought up Catholic and had never even considered the question of abortion; I just accepted that it was wrong. Now, I was thinking about it because I couldn't begin to think how to tell Jake that I was pregnant with somebody else's baby and I didn't even know who! And our parents would just flip out.

Abortion wasn't a service provided at the college infirmary, so the nurse referred me to a private doctor who did them. I went for the appointment and the doctor was nice and understanding. He examined me (very embarrassing) and said that I was just about eight weeks along and the abortion would be a simple procedure. He told me all about it and then we made an appointment for me to have it done the following Monday (it was a Friday when I saw him.)

I cried all day Saturday and on Sunday, I realized that I just had to talk with Jake about all of this. If we loved each other so much we could handle my being honest about this. I called him at home where he was recuperating and we had a long talk. I know he had trouble understanding me at times because I was crying so hard. Jake is so wonderful – he said that this wasn't my fault; obviously, I had been drugged and was raped. That was the first time I really knew that I should call it that. He said that he loved me and he would love any baby that I had and that raising the baby would make it his. Then he hung up to talk with his parents about all this and they ended up phoning my parents, who went right over to Jake's house. Then they called me – parents on each extension phone – and we all laughed and cried together. I didn't go for the abortion. The following weekend, Jake and I went to the Justice of the Peace and got married and we plan a lovely reception over the Christmas holidays. I took the next semester off and then transferred to be at the same college with Jake and our parents helped us with childcare. We are now the parents of a beautiful little girl, named Grace because she brought grace into our lives.

L

Laminaria tents – small rods of seaweed, also known as hydrophilic dilators, which are placed by a health professional into the cervix of a woman planned to undergo a surgical abortion. The material slowly absorbs moisture from the cervical canal and expands dilating the canal in the process. Other devices with similar hydrophilic (water-attracting) properties have been used for the same purpose. Laminaria tents may take a few days to act and these mechanical methods of cervical dilatation have now largely been replaced by the use of misoprostol placed vaginally.

Louisiana – rated F by **NARAL**. Louisiana has an unconstitutional and unenforceable ban on abortion by anyone other than the woman herself unless the abortion is necessary to preserve the woman's life or the pregnancy is the result of rape or incest reported according to stated requirements. The state code of Louisiana includes its intent to oppose and restrict reproductive choice. Louisiana has a law, enacted 6/17/2006, prohibiting abortion at any stage of pregnancy, from fertilization to birth, except in cases in which the mother's life is endangered. It also amended the criminal code on 6/02/06 to allow an 'unborn child' to be considered the victim of a crime independently of the pregnant woman. No abortion may be legally performed after viability unless to preserve the life or health of the woman. In such case, specific requirements exist to protect the wellbeing of the viable fetus. No public employee of Louisiana or any organization receiving state funds may recommend an abortion to a woman unless the employee is a physician who states that the abortion is necessary to preserve the woman's life. Public facilities may not be used to offer abortion services. Louisiana has an unconstitutional and unenforceable requirement that the husband of a married minor woman must give written consent before she can obtain an abortion. At least 24 hours before having an abortion, a woman must receive in person counseling about the procedure to be used, the gestational age of the fetus and her right to have all attempts made to preserve the life of the fetus if the fetus is 24 weeks of age or greater, a description of the fetus at the current gestational age and the risks associated with the abortion and with carrying a fetus to term. She must also receive state-prepared materials. Only physicians are allowed to perform legal abortions in Louisiana and these physicians are subject to a variety of requirements and restrictions not imposed on other physicians doing other procedures. All healthcare personnel and social service personnel may refuse to perform any service related to abortion without fear of legal reprisal. Public funding for abortion is prohibited except to preserve the life of the woman or when the pregnancy is the result of rape or incest. Minor women under 18 must have the notarized written consent of one parent prior to obtaining an abortion. This may only be waived in case of medical emergency or by judicial order.

Lowry, Shannon – receptionist at Boston, MA women's health clinic. Killed in 1994 by John Salvi. Salvi was found to be insane and committed suicide while in jail.

M

Mariam

My family is Middle Eastern and we run a grocery store in a small coastal city. Five years ago, when I was eighteen, my parents arranged for me to marry Sayeed, the son of a family friend. Children came quickly and now I have three little ones. They are aged one year old, two and a half, and almost four. Just before the baby was born, Sayeed said to me that he had fallen in love with a woman he works with and that he was leaving. He said he would give me the divorce. His parents and mine talked and Sayeed came back for a short time – just enough for me to get pregnant again. Four babies! Eeah! Then he left for good and is living with that woman now.

Me, I had to go back with my parents to work in the grocery and to live up top. It is hard and I was so tired. We all live over the shop, my mother, my father and my grandmother together with me and my children. There is no quiet place. I began to feel more and more depressed and not very well in myself. I felt like I was a baby machine. My mother is so good; she said to me that it is not forbidden to have an abortion this early in a pregnancy and she took me to the clinic to speak with the kind people there. There was a woman doctor who is of my religion and she was most kind and helpful. She talked with me of all the ways to do this and what might happen with each of them. I decided to take the pills because it could be so private – just my mother and me would know. I took the pills there in the clinic (and there was no bill because it is a charity sort of place) and then went home with my mother to look after me. It is best to keep these women things to ourselves.

Everything went easily and I recovered fast. I am happy that this choice was available to me; I have worries enough with Sayeed gone and the children to raise. I hope he really does give me the divorce and I can perhaps find another man to care for me and the children.

Maine – rated A by **NARAL**. State law ensures women's rights to pre-viability abortion. It requires that a woman be counseled by her physician of the 1) gestational age of the fetus, 2) the proposed abortion procedure and any risks involved and if she desires, information about alternatives to abortion and about resources available to provide her with assistance should she opt against abortion. Public funding for abortion is restricted to those cases in which the mother's life is endangered or the pregnancy is the result of rape or incest. Written consent by a parent or other adult family member is required for any woman under the age of 18. No abortion may be performed after a fetus is viable unless it be to preserve the mother's life. Maine allows pharmacists to dispense emergency contraception directly to women without a prescription. It also mandates that insurance plans that cover prescription drugs must provide equitable coverage for contraception. Maine law protects against violence directed at clinics.

Malta – abortion is completely forbidden by law and is not available even to save the life of the woman .As a consequence Maltese women are increasingly traveling abroad particularly to Spain to obtain legal abortion.

Manual vacuum extraction – a technique in which a narrow plastic tube or cannula is inserted into the uterus through the cervical opening and attached at the other end to a hand-operated vacuum pump in order to suction out the contents of the uterus. Because the tube is thinner than ones normally used with electrical vacuum suction, women find it more comfortable and less anesthesia may be needed than with suction curettage. This is a technique used to achieve abortion in early pregnancy, usually before seven weeks gestation, at which stage it has a lower failure rate than electrical suction curettage, around 1% as compared with nearly 3%. Also known as aspiration abortion.

Marie Stopes – see Stopes, Marie

Marie Stopes International World Wide – international organization with offices and clinics in 39 countries, devoted to improving women's reproductive health. MSIWW advocates for improvements in women's health as well as providing clinical services including contraceptive, sterilization and safe abortion services; the organization also trains health professionals in techniques related to women's reproductive health.

Maryland – rated A by **NARAL**. Maryland law ensures women's access to pre-viability abortion and to abortion at any stage in pregnancy if the woman's life or health are endangered or if the fetus is affected by a genetic defect or serious deformity or abnormality. Parental notification is required for women under 18 years of age unless the physician determines that the young woman to be in danger of physical or emotional abuse, of sufficient maturity to give informed consent, and that notification would not be in the best interests of the young woman. Abortion may be prohibited after viability unless necessary to preserve the mother's life or health or if the fetus is affected by a genetic defect or serious deformity or abnormality. Public funding may be used for a low-income woman's abortion only in cases of therapeutic abortion. Health insurance plans in Maryland are required to provide equitable coverage for any FDA approved contraceptives, if they provide coverage for prescription drugs.

Massachusetts – rated C+ by **NARAL.** Has not repealed its pre-Roe ban on abortion. It is also illegal to advertise abortion services. Massachusetts law requires that a woman receive specified counseling at least 24 hours before an abortion. This law has been challenged and found unconstitutional. The Massachusetts Declaration of Rights protects the right to reproductive choice as a fundamental right. The Massachusetts Supreme Court   has held that state medical assistance must be extended to medically necessary abortions. HMOs are not required to provide coverage for abortion services unless the abortion is necessary to preserve the woman's life. An unmarried woman under age 18 must obtain written consent of one parent. The law reads two parents, but this has been successfully challenged in the courts. Women eligible for state medical assistance have access to public funds to pay for medically necessary abortion or if the woman is a victim of rape or incest which has been reported to a law enforcement agency or public health agency within 60 days of the incident. Massachusetts law restricts abortion after 24 weeks gestation to those necessary to protect the mother's life or against "grave impairment" to her physical or mental health. Massachusetts law protects against clinic violence. Massachusetts law requires all insurance plans providing coverage for prescription drugs to provide equitable coverage for any FDA approved contraception. Emergency contraception requires a doctor's prescription. 79% of Massachusetts counties have an abortion provider.

Masturbation – self-stimulation of the genitals for sexual gratification. Sometimes suggested as an alternative to sexual intercourse as a means of birth control.

Maternity – the state of being a mother or pregnant.

Maturation – the process of attaining full development.

Mature – fully developed, or to attain full development.

Medical abortion – abortion caused by the use of drugs. See entries under **gemeprost, methotrexate, mifepristone, misoprostol.** The drugs are administered by a physician or a nurse acting under the direction of a physician. Drugs may be used individually but more often are used in combination. Depending on which drugs are used abortion occurs within 24 hours to 2 weeks after the drugs are administered (for details see individual drug entries.) Medical abortion may be performed in early or late pregnancy. Early medical abortion refers to the practice of using regimens combining mifepristone or methotrexate with misoprostol up to 63 days (nine weeks) from the first day of the last menstrual period; it is important to confirm the gestation (length of the pregnancy) usually with ultrasound and to be certain that the pregnancy is not ectopic. These regimens have been available in France and other European countries since the late 1980s, the United Kingdom since 1990, the United Sates since 2000. Generally the first drug is given in a clinic or hospital setting and the misoprostol 1-3 days later. Misoprostol may be given in a clinic setting or the woman may be provided with drug to administer herself, orally or intra-vaginally, at home. In a small percentage of cases (2-5%) aspiration or surgical evacuation of the uterus (**D&C**) may be required to complete the abortion. – percentages for different drug regimens are given under individual entries. When medical abortion is performed in later pregnancy this is done in a hospital setting; again a combination of drugs, usually mifepristone plus gemeprost or misoprostol, may be used or either gemeprost or misoprostol may be used alone. Pain and bleeding are normal accompaniments of medical abortion both early and late; analgesics, support and counseling are required. Side effects of mifepristone/misoprostol abortion include nausea, vomiting and diarrhea. Heavy bleeding occurs in about 1% women, necessitating either suction curettage (vacuum aspiration), and a scraping of the uterus using instruments (curettage or D&C) or ergonovine. A very small number of women, around 1:500-1,000, will require a blood transfusion. Infection may occasionally occur after the abortion requiring treatment with antibiotics. Also known as **medical termination of pregnancy**.

Medical termination of pregnancy – abortion achieved by medical means.

Medical tests prior to abortion – Certain investigations and precautions are regarded as good medical practice associated with abortion. This list is graded by the strength of the recommendation based on clinical evidence, with A being the most highly indicated, B somewhat less so.

1   Each woman should be given antibiotics just prior to abortion to prevent subsequent infection (A) or be screened for possible lower genital tract infection (B). The recommended antibiotic regimen is 1 gm of metronidazole at the time of abortion, followed by 100 mg doxycycline twice daily for seven days; 1 gm of azithromycin may be given as a single dose instead of doxycycline.

2   The woman should be tested for her blood group and Rh status. If she is Rh negative, she should be given Rhogam following the abortion to prevent her being sensitized and having difficulties in subsequent pregnancies (A).

3   The woman's hemoglobin should be checked to be sure that she is not anemic (A). Other lab tests should be done only if indicated by her personal history. (B)

4   If a woman has not had a Pap smear within the past year, she should be offered that one be taken at the time of the procedure (A) or advised to have one in the near future (B).

5   While not a test, it is important that each woman receive contraceptive counseling at the time of abortion and leave the clinic with her method of choice.

Medicolegal – relates to overlapping aspects of medical matters and the law.

Medroxyprogesterone acetate – a synthetic progestin (progestagen) used as a long-acting injectable contraceptive. See also Depo-Provera.

Melasma gravidarum – brownish patches of increased pigmentation across the cheeks, nose and forehead in pregnancy. Usually but not always disappears after return to non-pregnant state.

Membranes – the placenta and other structures surrounding and protecting the developing fetus. These are more properly called the fetal membranes and supply nutrients, oxygen and both hormonal and immune antibodies from the mother to the fetus. They also serve the excretory functions of the fetus.

Men and abortion In the United Kingdom –a March, 2001 court case brought the position of men in abortion decisions into the public arena. Stephen Hone attempted to use the courts to prevent a woman with whom he had had a short relationship from terminating her pregnancy. UK law has been consistent on the position of men in relation to abortion. Men have no legal right to prevent or insist upon abortion. In the last thirty years, three cases have come before the courts. Each time, the case for the man having the right to prevent an abortion has been rejected. The recent case did not even consider the question of Hone's right to prevent the abortion.

According to the British specialist abortion provider **bpas**, a majority of men in the United Kingdom back women's choice on abortion. bpas find that 'Male partners of women requesting abortion are usually supportive, often attend the clinic appointment with their wives or girlfriends and want more information about how to help. Around two thirds of women attending bpas clinics are accompanied by a man – usually a partner, brother or other male.'

A street survey of 200 London men, commissioned by bpas showed that: 74% would support a wife or girlfriend's choice to have an abortion if she had an unwanted pregnancy; a further 13% were unsure whether they would or not. Just 11% (n 23) said they would not support her. 54% said they personally knew a woman who had had an abortion. 63% said they felt there was insufficient information for men about abortion.

For US involvement of men in abortion decisions and practice see individual state entries. The website www.menandabortion.com is designed to help men be involved in the abortion decision and supportive of their partners. Most pro-life groups have sections on their websites encouraging men to support the 'right-to-life.'

Menarche – the first menstrual period. This usually occurs around twelve years of age.

Menhennitt ruling – judicial ruling by Justice Menhennitt in Victoria, Australia in 1969 directing that abortion was legal if it 'was necessary to preserve the woman from a serious danger to her life or her physical or mental health, not being merely the normal dangers of pregnancy and childbirth.' This followed a case brought against a medical practitioner, Dr Davidson, who argued that he had acted in good faith and in the interests of the woman. The Menhennitt ruling in this case has been liberally interpreted in Victoria and other Australian states but the Offences Against the Persons Act is still part of Victorian criminal law.

Menstrual extraction – suction of the menstrual blood and any products of conception from the uterus by means of an airtight, hand-operated suction device. Although this is similar to a standard first trimester aspiration abortion, this technique was embraced by feminists prior to the legalization of abortion. Aspiration devices were obtained from laboratory or chemical supply catalogs and the directions were passed from one woman to the next. The 1992 book, *A Woman's Book of Choices* explained menstrual extraction in detail, including instructions on the construction of the Del-**M** extraction device. This technique and the Del-M device were developed in the 1970s by Carol Downer and Lorraine Rothman. It was heralded by feminists as a means for them to control inconvenient menses as well as deal with suspected pregnancy. Many argued that using this technique was not abortion because women did not yet know whether they were pregnant. In January, 2005, a bill was introduced in Congress (HB 1841) making it a class 6 felony for any health professional to perform menstrual extraction without first doing a pregnancy test. The bill was tabled in committee.

Menstruation – cyclic bleeding from the uterus due to the breakdown and shedding of the lining of the uterus when pregnancy has not occurred during that cycle.

Meperidine – a narcotic analgesic often used for the pain of labor or post-operative pain.

Method – a manner of performing an act. See also maneuver, procedure, technique.

Methods of contraception – ways in which pregnancy can be averted

    abstinence – avoidance of sexual intercourse

    barrier methods – any method employing a physical device to prevent the sperm from entering the cervical canal, e.g. condoms, diaphragms

    Billings method – a method of periodic abstinence from sexual intercourse utilizing changes in cervical mucus to determine the time of ovulation.

    rhythm method – a method of periodic abstinence based on estimated 'safe days' on the calendar. This method is based on the assumption of a regular, 28 day cycle and abstaining from intercourse for a few days before, during and after the time of ovulation.

hemorrhage following vaginal birth or cesarean section. Misoprostol is a synthetic prostaglandin and the 200μg tablets are used in a dosage of 600 to 800μg, intra-vaginally or orally. When used in conjunction with mifepristone for medical abortion, misoprostol softens and 'ripens' the cervix, allowing it to open, and causes the uterus to contract to expel its contents. Misoprostol can be used on its own to prepare the cervix for surgical abortion (suction curettage or dilatation and curettage.)

Although misoprostol used alone can bring about complete medical abortion, both early and late, it is most commonly used as an adjunct to other agents, such as mifeprostone or methotrexate because by itself, it may take a number of days to achieve abortion and higher doses may be needed, leading to more side effects. It is usually given after the other agents in order to trigger the uterus to expel its contents. When used alone, surgical means may be necessary to complete abortion in up to 10% of cases.

Side effects of misoprostol include nausea, vomiting, diarrhea, bowel cramping, dizziness and headache. Pain and bleeding are an integral part of the abortion process and so are not side effects. Adequate oral analgesics (painkillers) may be needed for pain relief. There is some evidence that when misoprostol is used and is not successful in achieving abortion, and the pregnancy continues, there is an increased incidence of birth defects.

Misoprostol is now widely used as an abortifacient by women in countries where abortion is illegal. This has resulted in a sharp decrease in abortion-related deaths in countries such as Brazil and Uruguay, since although use of the drug without medical supervision still carries some risks, these are significantly less than those of abortions performed by non-medically trained practitioners using instruments.

Mississippi – rated F by **NARAL.** Only 2% of Mississippi counties have an abortion provider. Mississippi has not repealed its pre-Roe ban on abortion and in 1997, enacted a ban outlawing all abortions performed after 12 weeks gestation. A woman may not obtain an abortion until at least 24 hours after the doctor, in person, informs her of the gestational age of the fetus, describes the risks associated with the proposed procedure and the risks of carrying the pregnancy to term, and tells her the name of the physician who will perform the abortion. In addition, she must be told that medical assistance benefits may be available to help her with prenatal care, childbirth and neonatal care, that the father is liable for child support even if he has offered to pay for the abortion, and that she has a right to review state-prepared materials that describe the 'unborn child' and list agencies that offer alternatives to abortion. These state-prepared materials offer color pictures of the characteristics of the fetus in two week gestational age increments and reiterate the risks and the availability of alternatives, including possible funding. No public funds may be used to provide facilities for abortion, except when the procedure is necessary to preserve the woman's life, or in cases of rape or incest, or when there is a fetal anomaly inconsistent with live birth. Public funding for abortion for low-income women is only available in cases in which the woman's life is endangered, there is a fetal malformation incompatible with live birth or the pregnancy is the result of rape or incest. A woman under 18 who has never married or left the care, custody or control of her parents, may not obtain an abortion without the written consent of both parents. Exceptions are made in case of divorce or absence, in which the written consent of one parent will suffice, or in cases of incest by the father, stepfather or adoptive father, in which case the consent of the mother is accepted

Roussel Uclaf (RU) led by Dr Etienne-Emile Baulieu. Clinical trials conducted in France and Switzerland 1981. Licensed for use in France 1988, United Kingdom 1991, United States 2000. Now available in most European countries, Russia, Israel, China, New Zealand, Tunisia and Turkey. Mifepristone can be used to induce menses before a period is missed or to cause abortion either early in pregnancy or in the second trimester. Mifepristone acts by causing the developing embryo/fetus and its placenta to separate from the lining of the uterus. It also causes the cervix to soften and the uterus to release prostaglandins which in turn cause the uterus to contract. When mifepristone is used for medical termination of pregnancy, it is usually given together with **misoprostol** or **gemeprost**. These drugs are synthetic prostaglandins and trigger the uterus to expel its contents. This usually leads to a completed abortion. Side effects of mifepristone are usually minor and include nausea, vomiting, diarrhea and headache. Cramping is an expected part of the abortion and not considered a side effect; because of the cramps, most women require some form of pain relief. Heavy bleeding occurs in about 1% women, necessitating either aspiration, a scraping of the uterus (curettage) and/or ergonovine. A very small number of women, around 1:500-1,000, will require a blood transfusion. Infection may occasionally occur after the abortion requiring treatment with antibiotics. Mifepristone also shows promise for various non-abortion purposes – it is proving useful in the treatment of fibroids, endometriosis and uterine and breast cancers as well as some meningiomas (a type of brain tumor).

Miller, Vernice – pro-choice leader and advocate of legal rights of poor blacks. Miller was Director of the Center for Constitutional Rights, a non-profit group organized in the 1960s to provide legal services for poor blacks and civil rights activists. In the 1980s, the Center filed pro-choice *amices* briefs with the Supreme Court. Miller has advocated abortion rights as part of a more comprehensive program addressing women's and children's health.

Minipill – a form of birth control pill containing only progestin and no estrogen.

Mini-abortion – see Menstrual extraction.

Minnesota – rated C by **NARAL.** The Minnesota Constitution protects reproductive choice as a fundamental right. The Minnesota Supreme Court struck down a law limiting state medical assistance for abortion to cases of life endangerment and reported rape and incest. A woman may not have an abortion until at least 24 hours after the doctor informs her of the probable gestational age of the 'unborn child' and describes the procedure and the risks of both abortion and of carrying the child to term. In addition, she must receive state-mandated information that 1) medical assistance benefits may be available for prenatal care, childbirth and neonatal care, 2) that the father is liable for child support even if he has offered to pay for the abortion, 3) that she has a right to review state-prepared materials that describe the 'unborn child' and 4) a list of agencies that offer alternatives to abortion and contain information on 'fetal pain.' A woman under the age of 18 may not obtain an abortion until at least 48 hours after written notice is provided to both parents. If the notice is sent by certified mail, the 48 hour period begins at noon on the next day providing scheduled mail delivery. Minnesota law protects against clinic violence.

Miscarriage – popular term for spontaneous abortion.

Misoprostol – a drug commonly used to treat stomach and duodenal ulcers, heartburn and dyspepsia. It is used **off-label** to induce abortion, to complete miscarriage, or to stop

Population in Mexico City that the US would no longer fund foreign organizations that provided, counseled, referred or advocated abortion. In 1985 funding for the International Planned Parenthood Foundation was suspended. In 1993 one of the first post-inauguration decisions by President Clinton was to repeal the Mexico City Policy. After President George W. Bush was elected in 2001 one of his first acts was to re-instate the Policy.

Michigan – rated F by **NARAL.** In 2004, Michigan passed the 'Legal Birth Definition Act' by means of a citizen's initiative in concert with the vote of the legislature. This ban defines birth as the moment when any part of the child emerges from the birth canal. It could be interpreted as making any abortion illegal, although the stated intent was to prevent abortion of viable fetuses. The ban makes no provision for medically necessary termination. State law provides that no woman may receive an abortion until at least 24 hours after having received specified counseling utilizing state-prepared materials that include a pamphlet on prenatal care and parenting, medically accurate descriptions with illustrations or photographs of the characteristics of the fetus in two-week increments, describe abortion procedures and risks, identify services available to help the woman should she decide to carry her pregnancy to term, and finally, information that abortion may cause some women 'depression, feelings of guilt, sleep disturbance, loss of interest in work or sex, or anger.' State-funded pregnancy prevention programs may not provide abortion counseling or referrals. Community colleges are prohibited from including abortion services in health insurance plans offered its employees or dependants, except in situations where the woman's life is endangered. Public funding for abortion for low income women is restricted to those cases in which the woman's life is endangered or the pregnancy is the result of rape or incest. A woman under the age of 18, who is not emancipated, may not obtain an abortion without the written consent of one parent. Michigan law protects against clinic violence.

Midwife – a person who assists a woman in childbirth. Many abortionists in the period of illegal abortion (1870-1970 approximately) in the United States and Europe were midwives. In the US particularly some members of the medical profession and the media promoted the idea of a 'midwife problem', blaming midwives alone for the deaths of women after illegal abortions and claiming that all midwives were 'dangerous.' The aim was to downplay the role of some physicians in the provision of abortions as well as generally to discredit midwives and attempt to eliminate them from the provision of care for women in childbirth.

     certified nurse midwife – a person formally trained in obstetrics, usually a registered nurse. This person will have physician backup and often provides services within a hospital setting.

     lay midwife – a person with no formal medical credentials or training in obstetrics. Historically, the local midwife may also have been the abortionist. Some states, e.g. New Hampshire, now have an intermediary category of certified lay midwife. This is a person who has satisfied certain educational requirements designed by the state to ensure an acceptable level of proficiency in the care of pregnant women and women in labor.

Mifeprex – trade name of mifepristone (**RU 486**) in the United States.

Mifepristone – a synthetic steroid that acts to block progesterone. Also known as **RU-486.** Developed in France in 1980 by a team of scientists working for the company

cervical mucus method – see **Billings method**

hormonal methods – any method of birth control that relies on the use of natural or synthetic hormones. This includes the birth control pill, patches, some IUDs, injectable hormones, such as DepoProvera, vaginal rings and implants.

implants – hormonally- impregnated silicone objects that are inserted under the skin and that liberate a measured amount of hormone into the bloodstream in a steady controlled dose.

intrauterine devices – an object placed in the cavity of the uterus, acting as a foreign body, to prevent a fertilized ovum (egg) from implanting in the uterus. May contain copper which has an additional contraceptive effect, or synthetic progestin-type hormone which maintains the lining of the uterus in a state unreceptive to a fertilized ovum; the latter also acts to inhibit the passage of sperm through the cervical canal and up into the Fallopian tube where fertilization normally takes place.

symptothermal method – a combination of the rhythm and the temperature methods of periodic abstinence.

temperature method – a system of periodic abstinence from sexual intercourse based on the observation of the small variations in body temperature occurring at the time of ovulation.

withdrawal – a not very reliable method of avoiding pregnancy by removing the penis from the vagina just before ejaculation.

Methotrexate – a drug commonly used to treat cancer or autoimmune diseases, but also used **off-label** to induce medical abortion up to about 9 weeks, gestational age. Methotrexate interferes with the implantation of the embryo in the endometrium. Methotrexate is usually used in conjunction with other drugs to bring about medical abortion, usually misoprostol administered 3-7 days after the methotrexate is given orally or by injection. Methotrexate has been shown to be as effective as mifepristone in bringing about early medical abortion (prior to 9 completed weeks of pregnancy) – in about 95% of cases complete expulsion of the pregnancy occurs when the methotrexate/misoprostol regimen is used. However, it takes longer to act than mifepristone and has more side-effects (nausea, vomiting, and diarrhea). Occasionally surgical evacuation of the uterus is required to complete the abortion. With the introduction of mifepristone the use of methotrexate for medical abortion has declined in the US and elsewhere. However during the 1990s well conducted trials showed it to be safe and effective for medical abortion.

Mexico – the access to legal abortion in Mexico varies from state to state. Most states allow abortion in cases of rape or when the woman's life is endangered. Some allow abortion when it is known that there are severe birth defects in the fetus. In the State of Yucatan abortion is allowed when the pregnancy would result in grave economic difficulties and the woman already has three or more children. There is confusion and lack of understanding of the laws, resulting in 106,620 hospitalizations in Mexico every year because of the complications of unsafe abortions (source: Alan Guttmacher Institute) 23% of Mexican pregnancies are unwanted and 17% result in abortion. Abortion is the third or fourth cause of maternal mortality in Mexico (varying from year to year) The government health agencies offer only two methods of contraception: the IUD and sterilization.

Mexico City Policy – Decision announced at the UN International Conference on

Missouri – rated F by **NARAL.** Bans abortion after twelve weeks; this has been held unconstitutional because it provides no exception to protect a woman's health. In 2003, a law was enacted prohibiting a woman from obtaining an abortion until at least 24 hours after the treating physician had conferred with her and discussed 'the indications and contraindications, and risk factors including any physical, psychological, or situational factors for the proposed procedure and the use of medications, including but not limited to mifepristone, in light of her medical history and medical condition.' This law has been enjoined by a federal court. No public funds may be used to provide abortion counseling unless the woman's life is endangered. Health insurance policies in the state of Missouri must exclude coverage for abortion for any reason other than to preserve the woman's life. Missouri law states that: 'It is the intention of the general assembly of the state of Missouri to grant the right to life to all humans, born and unborn, and to regulate abortion to the full extent permitted by the Constitution of the United States, decisions of the United States Supreme Court, and federal statutes.' In addition, 'the general assembly of this state finds that: 1) the life of each human being begins at conception; 2) Unborn children have protectable interests in life, health and well-being, and the laws of this state shall be interpreted and construed to acknowledge on behalf of the unborn child at every stage of development, all the rights, privileges, and immunities available to other persons, citizens, and residents of this state.' A public facility may not be used for performing, assisting in or counseling an abortion unless the woman is endangered of her life. A public employee may not, within the scope of his employment, participate in an abortion unless it is necessary to save the woman's life. Missouri law prohibits public funding of abortion for low-income women unless the attending physician attests that the woman's life is endangered by a physical condition caused by or arising from the pregnancy or that the pregnancy is the result of rape or incest. A woman under the age of 18 may not obtain an abortion without the written consent of one parent. Missouri law requires that health insurance plans that provide coverage for prescription drugs also provide equitable coverage for FDA approved contraception.

MMR –Mortality Rate, Maternal

Moody, Howard – New York clergyman who in 1967, together with other clergymen set up a telephone counseling and referral service for pregnant women in need, giving them the names of illegal, but safe, abortionists. This was called the Clergyman Consultation Service.

Mole – see Hydatidiform mole

Molly Blythe – author of 'mollysavestheday' blog.

MollySavesTheDay.blogspot.com – a blog by a feminist author who has posted instructions on how to perform an abortion on oneself or a friend as a response to the South Dakota ban on abortion.

Montana – rated A- by **NARAL.** The Montana Constitution protects the right to reproductive choice as a fundamental right. A Montana court struck down a regulation limiting state medical assistance for abortion to cases of life endangerment, rape and incest. The court also struck down provisions requiring parental notice or judicial waiver before a minor could obtain an abortion. Montana provides that post-viability abortions may only be done to preserve the life or health of the mother and that certification of this by two doctors is required. At least 24 hours prior to an abortion, the attending physician must counsel the woman about 1) the probable gestational age of the fetus, 2) the risks associated with the proposed procedure and 3) the risks associated with carrying the pregnancy to term. She must also receive from the doctor or his agent a state-mandated lecture stating that 1) medical assistance may be available for prenatal care, childbirth and neonatal care, 2) that the father is liable for child support even if he has offered to pay for an abortion, and 3) that she has the right to review state-prepared materials that illustrate the characteristics of the unborn child at two week increments of gestational age, reiterate the methods and risks of abortion procedures, and provide resources for alternatives to abortion.

Morbidity – disease; also, the percentage of a given population that has a specific disease at any given time.

Morgentaler, Henry – Montreal doctor who challenged the 1969 abortion law that limited a woman's access to abortion. The inability of the government to get a jury to convict him led to the law being declared unenforceable and the law was ultimately found unconstitutional by the Supreme Court of Canada.

Morning-after pill – see Contraception, emergency

Mortality – condition of being mortal; also, the number of deaths at a particular time or a percentage of the population dying from a given condition.

Mortality Rate, Maternal– the number of women dying during or shortly after pregnancy, from causes related to the pregnancy, usually expressed as the Maternal Mortality Rate (MMR) for a given population. The World Health Organization in 1992 defined a maternal death as 'the death of a woman while pregnant or within 42 days of delivery, miscarriage or termination of pregnancy, from any cause related to or aggravated by the pregnancy or its management, but not from incidental or accidental causes.' In developed countries the maternal mortality is calculated per 100,000 live births or per 100,000 maternities (number of live births at any period of pregnancy plus stillbirths of 24 weeks or later) and figures of around 10-13 deaths per 100,000 maternities are usual. Most recent figures for the United States are around 12 deaths per 100,000 births. Reasonably accurate figures for MMR are available from 1850 for European countries, 1880 for Australia and New Zealand and 1900 for the United States. Rates fell steadily during the period up to 1950 from levels of 500-1000 deaths per 100,000 births to less than 200 per 100,000 births. During the first four decades of the 20th century however the US experienced one of the highest MMRs in the developed world – around 700 deaths per 100,000 births – 30 times today's figures. Rates in Europe were around 300-450 deaths per 100,000 births at the time. One of the important factors contributing to these deaths in women was the practice of illegal abortion.

In the years following the legalization of abortion in developed countries MMRs dropped dramatically. In New York City, the MMR dropped 45% in the year following the legalization of abortion in the state. In the United Kingdom the rate fell to the most recent figure of 12 per 100,000 maternities.

In less developed countries MMRs similar to those of early 20th century Europe and America continue to be the norm. WHO has estimated that the world MMR is 400 deaths per 100,000 births or 1600 women dying each day around the world; 99% of these deaths are in under-developed countries where a woman's overall chances of dying from a complication of pregnancy or childbirth are 200 times those of women in developed countries. WHO lists five main causes of maternal death: abortion is one of these. While complications of spontaneous abortion may contribute to these deaths the main cause is illegal induced abortion and its sequelae. Women's lifetime risk of dying due to maternal causes (pregnancy and childbirth and related causes) are: in Africa 1:20, in Asia 1:94, in Latin America 1: 160, in the United Kingdom 1: 5100.

In 2005 the Centers for Disease Control reported that 'the annual maternal mortality rate from legal abortion is extremely low,' adding that 'improving women's access to early abortion services such as medical abortion may further reduce the mortality rate.'

reproductive mortality – the sum of the deaths related to pregnancy and those caused by any contraceptive method or device.

Mucus – a slippery mixture of exfoliated cells, mucin, water and salts. It is secreted by mucus membranes to lubricate and protect them.

cervical mucus – secreted by glands in the cervical canal. The consistency of this mucus varies with hormonal influences. Early in the menstrual cycle, under the influence of estrogen, the mucus is thin. It gets thinner and more elastic just before ovulation and thickens and gets very sticky after ovulation. In pregnancy, the mucus is very thick and forms a plug in the cervix.

Multigravida – woman who has been pregnant more than once.

Multipara – a woman who has carried at least two babies to a viable gestational age.

N

Nancy

Elsa, a patient of Michele's told the following story as it was told by her grandmother: We lived on the family farm, the one Mother took over when Papa died so tragically young. There were six of us and we all worked hard to keep our farm and happy home going. I was eight when Nancy was born and her birth was just a few months after we buried Papa, so she was a balm to our sorrow.

Mother's system in raising this large family alone was that each child was the caretaker of the next youngest; hence, I cared for Nancy and saw her grow and flower into a lovely young woman.

Her special gift was to hear music in the soughing of the wind through the leaves, the rustle of autumn foliage, the twitter of birds and the lowing of cows. We would often, when chores were done for a few hours, take our sewing and a wrapped lunch down to the meadow under the trees by the river. There Nancy would dance to the tunes that ran through her head. Her hair of gilded russet would stream out around her like ribbons and her skirt would skirl with the silent music.

When Nancy was seventeen, our little community of farm families called a minister to preach to us about the word of God. We could give him a living of rotating among our homes and eating at our tables, but little else. Of course, a young novice preacher was sent to us. Many of the young women found his looks pleasing and I saw our Nancy cut the keen glance his way at table. We were all busy, as we always are in the summer, when we must secure the food and fuel for the bitter winter months and I suspect we were a bit negligent, not suspecting that a man of the cloth could betray a young girl's honor and innocence.

In September, just before the preacher was to move on to his next abode, Nancy told me that they loved each other. I said he needed to do the honorable thing and speak to our mother and eldest brother, Ben. She said he planned to return to do so.

Over the next month, Nancy seemed to droop like a daisy with no rain. She became quieter and quieter and spent many hours down by the river. A chill was coming in the air and I worried for her health. The bloom was gone from her cheeks and she ate no more than would sustain a kitten.

The week leading to Thanksgiving, a glow came on Nancy's cheeks and the spirit back into her eyes; Mother had a letter from the preacher saying that he would take the Thanksgiving feast with our family.

The day came and the meal and it was fine and good fellowship was enjoyed by all, but no words from the preacher to Mother or Ben. Nancy slipped to the mud room with the preacher and when she returned (he having left), her face was white and her eyes looked suddenly hollowed. She soon excused herself to bed.

Nancy didn't come to dinner the next day. She had been very quiet at breakfast, but we had become accustomed to her quiet ways since summer and didn't remark it. After lunch and no sign of her, we searched. I went to see if she had slipped up to bed and found the empty packets of savin and pennyroyal and had so the first intimation of what was wrong.

Ben and I found her under the trees by the river. Her form was like a doll, carelessly flung upon the ground and the red bloom was like a sunset shadow of her skirt. Ben lifted her tenderly and carried her to Mother, whose heartbroken shrill sounds in my dreams still.

N

NARAL Pro-choice America – formerly known as the National Abortion and Reproductive Rights Action League (NARAL), founded in 1969 by Betty Friedan, Bernard Nathanson and Larry Lader as the National Association for the Repeal of Abortion Laws to promote the legalization of abortion. In 1973, after Roe vs. Wade, it became the National Abortion Rights Action League, then National Abortion and Reproductive Rights Action League. This non-partisan, non-profit organization lobbies for increased abortion and reproductive rights, supporting pro-choice lawmakers and political candidates, engaging in lawsuits, sponsoring events, and organizing members to contact their individual Congressmen to support pro-choice legislation. It also is involved with public sex education and other areas of women's reproductive rights.

NARAL ratings – see the individual US States' listings.

Narcotic – drug that relieves pain and produces sedation.

Natal – relating to birth.

Natality – birth rate.

National Abortion Federation –body providing pregnancy information, counseling and guidance to abortion services in North America.

National Health Service – the publicly funded health care service provided throughout England, Scotland, Wales and Northern Ireland

National Organization for Women – organization founded in 1966 by Betty Friedan and others, with an agenda of women's issues, involving restructuring traditional institutions including the family, marriage, childrearing and education. In 1967 NOW took on abortion as one of its main programs and sponsored numerous pro-choice initiatives.

National Right to Life Committee – founded in 1973 to oppose legalized abortion. Active in all anti-abortion campaigns. Instrumental in the 'Unborn Victims of Violence Act' which was initially introduced as a bill in Congress in 1999 and ultimately became law in 2003.

Nausea – the feeling that one needs to vomit.

Nauseate – to produce nausea.

Nauseous – relating to nausea.

Navel – the umbilicus.

Necrotic – relating to dead cells or tissue.

Neisseria gonorrhoeae – a bacterium causing the sexually transmitted disease, gonorrhea.

Neonatal – refers to the first four-six weeks after birth.

Neonate – from birth through the first 28-42 days of life.

Nebraska – rated F by **NARAL**. Nebraska has never repealed its pre-Roe anti-abortion ban; in addition, it has added to its laws language affirming the intent of the state to oppose abortion. Nebraska law mandates pre-abortion counseling that conforms to state guidelines and mandates a delay of at least 24 hours after the completion of counseling before an abortion can be performed. Nebraska prohibits state employees or healthcare organizations receiving state funds from counseling women about abortion or referring them to abortion providers or counselors. No insurance or HMO wholly or partly funded with public monies can cover abortion services, except when the woman's life is endangered. Abortion coverage is available only as a special rider to policies and only of the individual bears all costs. Only physicians may legally perform abortions in Nebraska. Under Nebraska law, no individual or institution may be forced to provide abortion services; all healthcare personnel and institutions may refuse these services without jeopardy. They are required to inform the woman of their policy and they have no legal obligation to refer the woman elsewhere or to provide information or other reproductive services. Women eligible for state medical assistance have no access to abortion unless the pregnancy endangers their life or is the result of rape or incest. Nebraska also prohibits the use of federal funds for abortion services, but this is in conflict with federal law. One parent of an unemancipated woman under 18 must receive written notice at least 48 hours before an abortion may be performed. This may be waived if the physician attests that continuation of the pregnancy poses a grave risk to the young woman's life or health or if the woman notifies the proper authorities that she is a victim rape, incest or abuse.

Netherlands, The – Abortion legal and provided free of charge to Dutch citizens and foreign residents; the Netherlands has also been a common destination for women from abroad who have difficulty accessing abortion in their own countries, although the number of non-residents having abortions has fallen steadily since the mid-1980s. A woman requesting an abortion in the Netherlands is required to have a consultation with a physician, who may be the physician providing the abortion, and there is a 5 day **'cooling-off' period** between the date of this consultation and the date on which the abortion is performed; abortion on demand is available up to 23 weeks gestation. The abortion rate in the Netherlands is one of the lowest in the world (at around 5-6 abortions per thousand women per year); this is believed to be because great emphasis is placed on effective contraception and on adequate and non-judgmental sex education in schools.

Nevada – rated A- by **NARAL**. Nevada has an affirmative right-to-choice law. In Nevada, legal abortion can only be performed by physicians and there are special regulations applied to abortion that are not applied to other procedures, for example, that abortions be performed only in hospitals or specialized facilities. Nurses, nursing assistants and other employees hired to provide direct personal care to patients may not be required to participate in abortion-related services by their employer if they have notified the employer in writing of their personal moral, religious or ethical reasons for not doing so. These personnel are not exempted from care for the patient in a medical emergency. Similarly, private hospitals and clinics may refuse to provide abortion services. The use of public funds for abortion services are prohibited unless the abortion is necessary to save the life of the woman, or in cases where the pregnancy is the result of rape or incest and the woman has formally attested to this. Nevada law requires parental notification of one parent of any unemancipated woman under 18. This law has been found unconstitutional and unenforceable by a federal court because it does not sufficiently protect a young woman's constitutional right to an abortion because the judicial bypass provided for under the law is inadequate to protect the woman's rights. Nevada law protects against clinic obstruction or violence. Nevada law requires all insurance plans covering prescription drugs to provide equitable coverage for contraception. Nevada requires a specific informed consent for abortion: the woman must be informed of how many weeks pregnant she is, the procedure must be explained thoroughly, including any possible physical or emotional sequelae. Nevada restricts abortion after the 24th week of pregnancy to those cases where there is grave danger to the mother's physical or mental health.

New Hampshire – rated B+ by **NARAL.** New Hampshire law requires that insurance plans that cover prescription drugs provide equitable coverage for contraception. New Hampshire law allows pharmacists to provide emergency contraception directly to women without a prescription. Public funding may not be used for abortion services in New Hampshire unless the procedure is necessary to preserve the woman's life or the pregnancy is the result of rape or incest. As of March 2007, New Hampshire law no longer requires that one parent of an unemancipated woman under the age of 18 must be notified at least 48 hours prior to the abortion.

New Jersey – rated B by **NARAL.** The New Jersey state constitution provides greater protection for a woman's right to choose than does the federal constitution. New Jersey has an unconstitutional and unenforceable ban on abortion as early as twelve weeks; a permanent injunction was placed against enforcement of this ban because it is too vague and constitutes an undue burden on a woman's right to choice. New Jersey permits only physicians to perform abortion and imposes special restriction and conditions on abortion that are not imposed on other procedures. New Jersey provides that no health care personnel or institutions may be required to perform abortion services; this has been found unconstitutional as applied to non-sectarian, non-profit hospitals, which can not prohibit the use of their facilities for first trimester abortion. New Jersey law requires notification of at least one parent of an unemancipated woman under the age of 18 at least 48 hours before an abortion procedure can be done. This law has been found unconstitutional and unenforceable by a New Jersey court because it violates the state constitution's equal protection provision. New Jersey law provides that all insurance plans that provide prescription drug coverage must provide equitable coverage for contraception; there is, however, a refusal clause applying to religious employers for whom contraceptive practices are contrary to their established religious beliefs and practices. The right of refusal applies to sterilization procedures in the same way as to abortion. New Jersey mandates that hospitals providing emergency care for rape victims must provide access to emergency contraception. New Jersey allows state medical funds to be used for medically necessary abortions. In determining medical necessity the following factors are acceptable: whether the abortion is necessary to preserve the life of the mother; whether the pregnancy is the result of rape or incest; physical, psychological and emotional factors; age and family reasons. 90% of New Jersey counties have an abortion provider.

New Mexico – rated B+ by **NARAL.** New Mexico's state constitution provides more protection than the federal constitution for a woman's right to choose. The New Mexico legislature has passed a pro-choice resolution. New Mexico has not repealed its pre-Roe unconstitutional and unenforceable ban on abortion. Only physicians are allowed to perform legal abortions in New Mexico. New Mexico law allows any hospital or it employees or staff to refuse to provide abortion services on the basis of moral or religious reasons. New Mexico has an unconstitutional and unenforceable requirement for the consent of one parent before any minor woman under the age of 18 can have an abortion.

It does not require a constitutionally required judicial bypass procedure. New Mexico allows state funds to be used for abortion if 1) the procedure is necessary to preserve the woman's life, 2) the pregnancy has been certified the result of incest or rape, 3) the procedure is necessary to terminate an ectopic pregnancy, 4) the procedure is medically necessary because pregnancy aggravates a pre-existing condition, makes treatment impossible, interferes with diagnosis, or has an otherwise profound negative effect on the woman's physical or mental health. New Mexico law requires all insurance plans that provide prescription drug coverage to provide the same coverage for contraception; religious employers are exempted. In New Mexico, pharmacists are allowed to provide emergency contraception without a prescription. New Mexico law makes the performance of any post-viability procedure a felony unless the procedure is necessary to preserve the life of the mother or to prevent great bodily harm to the woman.

New South Wales – The Crimes Act 1900 (NSW) establishes criminality for inducing an abortion, including for the woman herself, in sections 82, 83 and 84. There is no defence to the sections, other than the interpretation of what is 'lawful'. In 1971 in a case brought against Dr Wald, Justice Levine determined that abortions in NSW are lawful where 'the operation was necessary to preserve the woman involved from serious danger to her life or physical or mental health which the continuance of the pregnancy would entail' and the treating doctor may take in to account 'the effects of economic or social stress that may be pertaining to the time'. There have been no further attempts at prosecution of doctors performing abortions since this case.

With the eventual introduction of mifepristone in New South Wales, changes in the wording of the law to cover medical abortion may be necessary. Under section 82 there are penalties for a woman who 'unlawfully administers to herself' substances to induce abortion. While mifepristone is administered to a woman in a hospital or clinic, misoprostol which is the second drug required in the process, can be safely administered by the woman herself at home. However it seems likely that where mifepristone and misoprostol have been lawfully prescribed to the woman, if she administers misoprostol to herself, it will not contravene section 82.

In practice surgical abortion is widely available in NSW cities but less accessible in rural areas. Most surgical abortions are performed in free-standing clinics and only a few early abortions in hospitals. Late abortion for fetal abnormality is available in both public and certain private hospitals. Medical abortion using methotrexate and/or misoprostol is available from individual doctors and some clinics.

New York – rated A- by **NARAL**. New York requires that only physicians perform legal abortions and has specific restrictions and requirements for abortion that it does not have for other procedures. Individuals and hospitals may refuse to participate in abortion services based on conscience or religious grounds. Individuals must present their refusal in writing and state the reasons for so refusing. Hospitals must inform the patient of appropriate resources. New York State allows state funds to be used for abortion when medically necessary. The definition of 'medically necessary' is very broad. Any insurance plan in New York State that covers prescription drugs must provide equitable coverage for contraception; an exception can be made for religious employers. New York law requires that sexual assault victims be offered emergency contraception in hospital emergency rooms. New York protects against clinic obstruction or violence. New York law prohibits abortion after 24 weeks except when necessary to preserve the woman's life. It also requires that when any abortion is performed after 20 weeks, a second physician be present to provide care to any live birth.

New Zealand – both surgical and medical abortion are available in New Zealand although to date medical abortion has been confined to larger centers.

The Contraception, Sterilization, and Abortion Act 1977 set up the Abortion Supervisory Committee which reports annually to Parliament. This Act restricts where abortions may be performed. For pregnancies under 12 weeks abortions may be carried out in a licensed clinic and for pregnancies over 12 weeks abortion must be carried out in a licensed hospital. The Act defines the type of licenses for premises and the Abortion Supervisory Committee issues the licenses.

The Abortion Supervisory Committee sets up and maintains the list of certifying consultants who may approve abortions and oversees services. Counseling services must be available.

A woman seeking an abortion must be referred by a doctor, usually a general practitioner or a family planning doctor, who will arrange a referral to a licensed clinic (for a pregnancy under 12 weeks) or to a specialist operating in a licensed hospital (for a pregnancy over 12 weeks).A woman seeking an abortion must obtain the approval of two certifying consultants, one of whom must have experience in obstetrics. A certificate must be issued for the performance of an abortion.

A doctor who has a conscientious objection to abortion is not required to assist in the performance of an abortion but the doctor has an obligation to refer the woman on for assessment if this is requested.

The grounds for an abortion are still subject to the Crimes Act 1961 (and amendments from 1977 and1978). These grounds are:

1   Serious danger to life
2   Serious danger to physical health
3   Serious danger to mental health
4   Any form of incest or sexual relations with a guardian
5   Mental subnormality
6   Fetal abnormality (added in the July 1978 amendment)

In addition, other factors which are not grounds in themselves but which may be taken into account are:

1   Extremes of age
2   Sexual violation (previously rape)

Self-abortion is an offence.

Since 2001 medical abortion using mifepristone/misoprostol has been available in a small number of New Zealand clinics.

The New Zealand statistics on abortion are amongst the most detailed and comprehensive in the world. Between 1981 and 2000 nearly 250,000 abortions were performed in New Zealand with no maternal deaths.

NHS – see National Health Service

Nondisjunction – failure of paired chromosomes to separate properly during cell division, so that both chromosomes are received by one of the daughter cells and none by the other. This results in certain genetic abnormalities, most commonly, Down syndrome.

Nonparous – not having borne a child at longer than 20 weeks gestation.

Non-Steroidal Anti-Inflammatory Drugs – drugs such as ibuprofen and mefenamic acid which counteract the production of natural prostaglandins by the body. Prostaglandins cause painful contractions of the uterus during abortion procedures – NSAIDs in conjunction with other analgesics or anesthetics have been successful in reducing pain during surgical abortions. In one study of medical abortions ibuprofen was found to be associated with a slightly increased rate of failed abortions and therefore paracetamol/codeine combinations may be more appropriate analgesics.

Nonviable – not capable of life.

Nor-progestins – progestins commonly used in conjunction with estrogen as contraceptive, in oral, patch or vaginal form.

North Carolina – rated D by **NARAL**. Only physicians are allowed to perform legal abortions in North Carolina and special restrictions and requirements apply to abortions that do not apply to other procedures. Any healthcare provider in North Carolina may refuse to participate in abortion procedures on the basis of religious, moral or ethical reasons. The use of state funds for abortion is prohibited except when the life of the woman is endangered or when the pregnancy is the result of rape or incest. North Carolina restricts the access to abortion of minor women under the age of 18, who are not emancipated. It requires the consent of one parent, or if she has been living with a grandparent for more than six months, the grandparent. Consent may not be waived without court order unless a physician determines that there is a medical emergency requiring an immediate abortion. North Carolina law provides that any insurance plan providing prescription drug coverage also provide equitable coverage for contraception. It exempts religious employers from this requirement. North Carolina protects against clinic obstruction or violence. North Carolina prohibits abortion after 20 weeks unless the woman's life is endangered or continuance of the pregnancy would gravely impair her health.

North Dakota – rated F by **NARAL.** North Dakota has an unenforceable and unconstitutional ban on abortions performed as early as 12 weeks. This ban was enacted in 1999 and was found unconstitutional in 2000. It also has an Abortion Control Act, which expresses opposition to abortion and the intent to restrict the right to choose. In 2005, the North Dakota legislature passed a resolution declaring its opposition to a woman's right to choice. North Dakota has a law prohibiting any public funds, including federal monies, from being used by any family planning agency that performs or refers for abortion. This has been invalidated by a court. It further prohibits funds distributed by the Children's Services Coordinating Committee be used for direct referral of minors for abortion. A woman may not obtain an abortion until at least 24 hours after receiving mandatory counseling using state-prepared materials. North Dakota has an unenforceable and unconstitutional law requiring that any married woman have her husband's consent. Only physicians are allowed to perform legal abortions in North Dakota and there are unenforceable and unconstitutional restrictions on abortion providers that are not placed on other medical providers. By law, health insurance providers in North Dakota must exclude coverage for abortion unless it is necessary to preserve the woman's life. Abortion is prohibited in any state-owned facilities. No healthcare personnel or institutions are required to perform an abortion in North Dakota for any reason. North Dakota prohibits the use of public funding for abortion unless the woman's life is endangered or the pregnancy is the result of rape or incest. North Dakota requires that an unmarried woman under 18 have written consent from both parents before having an abortion. This may be waived only by court order. North Dakota prohibits abortion after the fetus 'may reasonably be expected to have reached viability' unless the attending physician and two consulting physicians attest that continuing the pregnancy would endanger the woman's life or impose a 'substantial risk of grave impairment of her physical or mental health.' It further provides that in these cases, a second physician must attend a post-viability abortion with the sole responsibility of caring for any live borne infant.

Northern Territory (Australia) – Abortion may be performed in the Northern Territory if the pregnancy is less than 14 weeks and 'continuation of the pregnancy involves greater risk to women's life or the risk of injury to physical or mental health than termination' It may also be performed later in pregnancy if serious physical or mental abnormalities are detected in the fetus. Abortion must be performed by a specialist gynecologist in a hospital which has effectively restricted the provision of surgical abortions to Darwin and Alice Springs hospitals.

NOW – National Organization for Women.

Nuchal – relating to the back of the neck.

Nuchal translucency testing – ultrasound measurement of the layer of fluid under the skin on the neck of the developing fetus, usually done between 11 and 14 weeks. An increased thickness may be associated with Down syndrome or other genetic deformities or some types of heart problems.

Nulligravida – woman who has never been pregnant.

Nullipara – woman who has never borne a baby at 20 weeks or longer gestation.

O

Olivia

It was 1970 and the Beatles were still big. I turned eighteen that summer and was enjoying a new-found freedom. It was the perfect summer: hot days and cool evenings, lazy days at the beach and a few hours work each evening as an usher at the movie theater. This was my last year in high school and I looked forward to being at the top of the pecking order and to the excitement of applying to colleges.

It was also the summer that I tried many new things, things that I thought were grown-up and daring. I tried cigarettes but didn't like them. Sweet alcoholic drinks were another matter; they tasted good and made me feel relaxed and drifty and happy to be with my friends. Last of all, just the week before school reopened, I tried sex. I didn't have a real boyfriend, a crowd of us all hung out together, but it just seemed like another fun thing that we could all do together. I sort of knew the connection between sex and baby-making, but thought it couldn't happen unless certain vague conditions were met and that it certainly couldn't happen to me.

One month into school, I began to feel sick all the time. At first, Mom and I thought it must be anxiety about the pressures of senior year, but Mom became alarmed when my weight loss became apparent. This triggered the first doctor's visit. Blood work was done and a physical exam, but no pregnancy test or pelvic exam. Dr. Evans asked me if I had a boyfriend and I answered no. All the tests were normal, so Dr. Evans suggested that perhaps it was just senior nerves and he gave me and Mom tips on how I should eat, in order to stop losing weight. He also said that I should come back for some tranquilizers if it continued.

Over the next month, the terrible queasiness subsided, to be replaced by a need to pee all the time. Another quick trip to Dr. Evans eliminated the possibility of a bladder infection.

At the end of the next month, even though I had maintained my weight loss at five pounds, I suddenly was unable to button my jeans. For the first few days, I just wore a long shirt, but I was beginning to have a little scared feeling that maybe I was pregnant. I was afraid to mention this to my mother – afraid both of Mom's reaction and also to make it real. By the end of that week, there was no choice. Mom noticed my little pot belly and immediately perceived the possibility. Another trip to Dr. Evans, and this time a definitive diagnosis. I was about four months pregnant.

On Sunday, my grandparents came to the house and conferred for hours with my parents and finally, I was called in to hear my future. The adults agreed that the best solution would be for me to go and live with Aunt Rita in California until after the baby was born. The parish priest would make arrangements with Catholic Charities in California for the adoption of the baby and after that I could finish my last year of school. I felt numb and like a bad child.

Twenty years later, after recurring nightmares in which my baby was snatched from my arms, over and over again, I decided to find the son I gave up. I was now an experienced teacher and mother of two more children, It was difficult but I felt that I could never have peace until I made the effort. After five years, I received a letter – the handwriting was strangely like my own – and was greeted by my son. He wanted to meet me and his adoptive parents encouraged him. He told me that he was very lucky: the parents who raised him were very loving and wonderful and had always told him that they had chosen him and that one day, he might want to meet the woman who gave him birth and had the great misfortune of being unable to raise him.

O

Obesity – excessive accumulation of fat in the body.

    morbid obesity – obesity severe enough to threaten health.

Obstetrician – a physician who specializes in pregnancy and childbirth.

Obstetrics – the medical specialty concerning itself with pregnancy and childbirth, both normal and complicated.

Octoxynol 9 – commonly used spermicide in barrier contraceptives.

Offences against the Persons Act – Bill passed in 1861 in Britain designed to protect women against unsafe practices intended to induce abortion in the pre-antibiotic era. The Act was in no way concerned with whether the woman was actually pregnant nor with the fetus. In Australia this Act became part of the Crimes Act of Victoria (1958) under which anyone found guilty of inducing an illegal abortion would be sentenced to jail for up to 15 years.

Off-label – using a drug which is licensed for one purpose for another, different medical purpose. This is a common and acceptable medical practice .When a drug company initially applies for a license for a drug a large amount of money usually has been invested in research, patent fees and the application process. If the drug is subsequently found to be useful for other purposes the company may be reluctant to dispense further funds on research and licensing when the drug is already in the marketplace. Physicians prescribing the drug for the 'off-label' purpose depend on what they know of its actions, side effects and risks from the medical literature and from colleagues. Most countries permit the use of 'off-label' drugs by the medical profession but require full disclosure by the physician to the patient. Misoprostol is currently licensed, in many countries where it is currently used, only for the treatment of gastric (stomach) ulcers despite the fact that it is known and widely used for many different obgyn indications including bleeding following childbirth or miscarriage, and for medical abortion in combination with mifepristone or methotrexate. Methotrexate when used with misoprostol for medical abortion is also used 'off-label.' The use of both these drugs 'off-label' is supported by a very large amount of scientific evidence as effective and safe.

Ohio – rated F by **NARAL**. Ohio bans some safe abortion procedures; it allows suction aspiration or curettage, and dilation and evacuation procedures. A woman may not have an abortion until at least 24 hours after receiving state-mandated counseling, using state-prepared materials. It prohibits the use of any state funds given to family planning services for abortion referrals or counseling. Ohio has unenforceable restrictions on the use of mifepristone. Only physicians are allowed to perform abortions in Ohio and they are subject to restriction not imposed on other medical providers. Any individual or hospital on Ohio may refuse to provide abortion-related services. State funds for insurance for state employees may not be used to provide abortion services unless necessary to preserve the woman's life or in cases of reported rape or incest. Individuals may obtain coverage by buying a rider to their policy at personal expense. Women receiving state medical aid can not use state funds for abortion unless the abortion is necessary to preserve the woman's life or the pregnancy is a result of rape or incest that has been reported through the designated agencies. A minor woman under the age of 18 who is not emancipated, married or in the armed services may not have an abortion without the written consent of one parent. The only exceptions are if there is an emergent medical need that endangers the life or physical health of the young woman or if she receives a court order. This law has been found enforceable. Ohio has an unconstitutional and unenforceable ban on post-viability abortion. It has been found unconstitutional because it is part of a pre-viability abortion ban that unduly burdens a woman's right to choose an abortion under federal law.

Oklahoma – rated D- by **NARAL**. Oklahoma has not repealed its pre-Roe criminal ban on abortion but it has amended the penalty portion of the law. Only physicians are allowed to perform legal abortions in Oklahoma and there exist unconstitutional and unenforceable restrictions on abortion providers that do not apply to other medical providers. A woman may not have an abortion until at least 24 hours after she has received state-mandated counseling, using state-prepared materials. By Oklahoma law, no healthcare professional or private hospital can be required to participate in the provision of abortion services; the exception is emergency medical aftercare of an abortion patient. Oklahoma prohibits the use of public funds for abortion services unless the life of the woman is endangered or the pregnancy is the result of rape or incest that has been reported to the appropriate authorities or the physician has certified that the woman is emotionally unable to so report. The law makes clear that if the federal government stops mandating funding of abortion in the cases of rape and incest, Oklahoma will stop covering these. Oklahoma has a post-viability ban, assuming 24 weeks to be the gestational age of viability. The only exception is if the abortion is necessary to preserve the life of the mother and stipulates that in those cases, the physician must use the method of abortion most likely to spare the life of the fetus and that a second physician must be in attendance to care for any live-born infant.

Oligohydramnios – deficient amniotic fluid; may signal death of the fetus, urinary abnormalities or intrauterine growth retardation.

Oligospermia – deficient number of sperm.

Onanism – coitus interruptus; an unreliable method of contraception.

Oocyte – ovum in the ovary.

Operation Rescue – militant anti-abortion activists

Opiate – any substance derived from opium, having pain-relieving and sedative properties.

Oregon – rated A- by **NARAL**. Oregon's state constitution provides more protection for a woman's right to choose than does the federal Constitution. Oregon law protects women and healthcare workers from clinic obstruction and violence. Oregon allows women eligible for state medical assistance to obtain public funds for abortion. In Oregon, no physician or other healthcare worker is required to counsel about or participate in abortion as long as he/she notifies the patient of this policy. Similarly, no private hospital is required to participate in abortion as long as they notify patients of their policies. A Sexual Assault Victims Emergency Medical Response Fund has been established by Oregon law and this fund pays for the medical assessment and care of sexual assault victims, including the offering and provision, when desired, of emergency contraception.

Orgasm – the culmination of the sexual experience, with involuntary contractions of the vagina and pelvic floor muscles in the woman and ejaculation of semen in the man.

Orifice – an opening into a body cavity.

Os – mouth or orifice.

        cervical os – the external opening of the cervix of the uterus into the vagina.

Outlet – a passage or opening that allows exit from the body.

Ovary – one of two paired organs in women that produce the eggs and hormones of reproduction.

Ovulation – the discharge of an ovum (egg) from the ovary.

Ovum – the egg or female reproductive cell.

Oxytocin – hormone produced by the hypothalamus that stimulates smooth muscle contraction, causing contraction of the pregnant uterus and ejection of milk from the breast.

P

Pauline

I'm over 50 now, widowed and living in Australia. I was married when I was 18, to Michael, he was the same age. We grew up together in a small town in the middle of Ireland. Back then, nobody talked about sex in Ireland, though everyone was trying it. There was no sex education in school and for me at least, none at home. I grew up knowing nothing at all about contraception. It was a constant struggle, boys were always on at you for sex but girls were supposed to say no at least until we were engaged. Getting pregnant outside marriage was the worst thing that could happen to a girl.

So when it happened to me our parents, both lots, insisted we get married – and soon. Of course everyone in the town knew what was happening but no-one would say it to your face. Then we had a honeymoon planned, ten days in Spain. We'd just got to Dublin Airport when I began to bleed, and I fainted. I came to in the ambulance on the way to hospital. I was having a miscarriage and the plane had gone without us.

In the hospital I cried and cried. The doctor said don't worry dear, it often happens the first time, you'll soon have another pregnancy and a beautiful baby. I wanted to say, that's not why I'm crying, it's because I got married when I didn't want to and now I don't need to be, but I just couldn't tell her that.

After that there was nothing left for Michael and me. We went to England and separated, though our families thought we were living together. When we were 21 we got divorced in England. A long time later I met Lew and married him, but I never got pregnant again. Talking about all this now makes me realize how many other women in those times were pushed into unhappy marriages just because of the social stigma of being pregnant.

P

Pain – physical or mental distress or suffering.

    fetal pain – There is good evidence that fetuses cannot experience pain before 22 weeks' gestation; the neural (nervous) circuitry for pain is immature and the developmental processes for the mindful experience of pain have not yet been completed.

    maternal pain – both surgical and medical abortion is usually accompanied by some degree of physical pain requiring pain relief – see Analgesia.

Parametritis – infection of the tissue around the uterus

Parenteral – introduced into the body by injection into or under the skin, into the muscles or directly into the circulation intravenously.

Parity – the state of having borne children.

Parous – having borne one or more children.

Partial-Birth Abortion Law – Partial birth abortion is defined as 'an abortion in which a physician deliberately and intentionally vaginally delivers a living, unborn child's body until either the entire baby's head is outside the body of the mother, or any part of the baby's trunk past the navel is outside the body of the mother and only the head remains inside the womb, for the purpose of performing an overt act (usually the puncturing of the back of the child's skull and removing the brain) that the person knows will kill the partially delivered infant, performs this act, and then completes delivery of the dead infant.' The language of the Act allows for no exception for medical necessity and states that this type of abortion is never medically necessary.

    The Partial Birth Abortion Ban Act (Public Law 108-105, HR 760, S 3) is the United States law that bans partial birth abortion. It was signed into law by George W. Bush on November 5, 2003. It was declared unconstitutional by federal judges in California, New York and Nebraska before it could be implemented. The Supreme Court ruled, in 2007, that the law is constitutional. The lower courts have held the law unconstitutional because it does not adequately protect the health of the mother. The law has never been enforced. **ACOG** opposes all State and Federal legislation known as the partial-birth abortion laws and has issued several Statements of Policy on the subject. ACOG believes such legislation to be 'inappropriate, ill-advised and dangerous,' having 'the potential to outlaw other abortion techniques that are critical to the lives and health of American women.'

Parturient – relating to childbirth.

Parturifacient – agent that induces labor.

Pathogen – disease-causing microorganism.

Pederasty – anal intercourse. Usually used to refer to man/boy.

Pelvic inflammatory disease (PID) – infection with bacteria, usually commencing in the cervix (often as a sexually transmitted infection but also following miscarriage, induced abortion or childbirth). May then progress to infection within the uterus (**endometritis**) and surrounding tissues (**parametritis**) and in the fallopian tubes (**salpingitis**). PID may be acute or chronic – chronic PID frequently follows an incompletely treated episode of acute PID and can be a cause on infertility. Acute PID can progress to septicemia if inadequately treated and may be fatal.

Pennsylvania – rated F by **NARAL**. In 1982, Pennsylvania enacted a statute expressing its intent to oppose abortion and restrict access to it in every way possible without violating federal law. Pennsylvania prohibits state employees or organizations receiving state funds from counseling or referring for abortion. A woman may not have an abortion until at least 24 hours after receiving a state-mandated lecture, using state-prepared materials; prior to this lecture, the physician must orally inform the woman of the probable gestational age of the fetus, the nature of the proposed procedure and any attendant risks and alternatives, and the medical risks of carrying the pregnancy to term. Pennsylvania has an unconstitutional requirement that the husband of any married woman be notified prior to her having an abortion. Pennsylvania restricts performance of legal abortions to physicians only, applying to these physicians restrictions not applied to other providers, and prohibits the use of state owned or operated healthcare facilities unless the procedure is necessary to preserve the life of the mother or the pregnancy is the result of rape or incest that has been reported to the appropriate authorities. No healthcare provider or employee of any health care facility can be required to participate in abortion related services as long as they have stated their objection in writing and it is based in religious, moral or professional reasons. Likewise, no hospital or health care facility can be required to participate in abortions against its stated policy. Health and disability insurance providers in Pennsylvania must offer a policy that expressly excludes coverage for abortion-related services except in cases where the woman's life is endangered or the pregnancy is the result of rape or incest. Health insurance plans for state employees may not cover abortion except then the woman's life is endangered or the pregnancy is the result of rape or incest that has been reported through the recognized channels. Similarly, women who are eligible for state medical assistance may not have an abortion funded by state monies unless the woman's life is endangered or the pregnancy is the result of rape or incest that has been reported by the woman herself to the appropriate authorities unless an independent physician certifies that the woman could not report the incident because of physical or psychological reasons. An injunction against the enforcement of the latter provisions exists because these provisions are in conflict with federal law. Pennsylvania law requires that any unemancipated woman under the age of 18 must obtain the permission of one parent. The only exceptions to this are if there exists a medical emergency requiring an immediate abortion to preserve the life of the woman or if any delay could cause serious risk of irreversible harm, or if the young woman can obtain court consent. Pennsylvania law prohibits any abortion after 23 weeks gestation unless the procedure is necessary to preserve the woman's life or prevent a substantial risk of irreversible harm. A provision that the physician must use the method of abortion least likely to cause harm to the fetus in these cases was found unconstitutional because it required the woman to bear an increased medical risk. A second physician must attend to care for any live-born infant.

Perforation – a hole made in an organ or tissue by disease or injury.

    cervical perforation – can be caused by surgical instruments used during therapeutic or diagnostic procedure, or by an intrauterine device extruding, or by sharp objects, such as knitting needles, used in the performance of illegal abortion.

    uterine perforation – the uterus can be perforated by instruments used to perform a surgical procedure or during the placement of an IUD.

Phytoestrogen – estrogen found in herbs (for example, black cohosh, dong quai, licorice) or other plants, such as soy or wild yams.

Pica – a craving for and ingestion of non-food substances, such as clay, which may occur during pregnancy. Sometimes, but not always, correlates with a mineral deficiency.

PID – see Pelvic inflammatory disease

Pile – common term for hemorrhoid. Often first experienced during pregnancy.

Pill, the – common term for oral contraception.

Placenta – the frisbee-shaped organ through which the fetus receives nourishment and excretes physiologic wastes. It is attached on one surface to the uterine wall and by the umbilical cord to the fetus.

     placenta accreta – a condition in which an abnormally attached placenta invades the wall of the uterus. This can cause hemorrhage after delivery (vaginal or caesarean) that may be life-threatening.

     low-lying placenta – a placenta that is placed low in the uterus, close to but not covering the inner opening of the cervix.

     placenta previa – the placenta is placed over or at the margin of the inner opening of the cervix; with dilatation of the cervix, the placenta can tear and cause massive bleeding. May be life-threatening for both the mother and the baby therefore delivery in cases of placenta previa is usually by cesarean section.

Planned Parenthood, International Federation for – an international organization, supporting reproductive health services for women, including provision of contraceptive information and supplies, sterilization procedures and abortion. In the US there are private clinics offering reproductive and preventive health care to women, including routine gynecological care, provision of contraceptive information and supplies, sterilization procedures and abortion.

Planned Parenthood of Australia – private clinics offering reproductive health services for men and women including abortion, sterilization procedures and provision of contraceptive advice.

Poland – from 1956 to 1990 abortion up to 12 weeks gestation was legal and freely available in Poland. In the early 1990s due to the intervention of the Catholic Church and with the support of physicians' groups the law became much more restrictive. In 1997 amendments to the Polish Abortion Act and to earlier 1993 legislation restricted abortion to situations where the mother's life or health was in danger (the diagnosis to be made by a physician not performing the abortion); to severe fetal abnormality (again, the diagnosis to be made by a physician not involved in performing the abortion) and to cases where the pregnancy is the result of a criminal act (the decision to be made by a state prosecutor.) As a result of this legislation the numbers of legal abortions performed in Poland are in the hundreds per year whereas it is estimated that 30,000-50,000 illegal abortions are performed annually in the country and that an unknown but large number of women go abroad each year for abortion.

Polyembryoma – a rare highly malignant tumor of germ cells, formed in the ovary or testis, that looks like a normal early embryo.

Polyhydramnios – excess amniotic fluid. Frequent in diabetic women.

Population Council – an international, non-governmental, non-profit organization that conducts research in the areas of social science, biomedical science and public health. It is committed to evaluating and developing sustainable means of enhancing the health and well-being of people, focusing on reproductive health, HIV/AIDS, poverty, gender and youth. The Council was established in 1952 by John D. Rockefeller III and currently has 18 offices in Africa, Asia and Latin America. While today lauded as a force for good, there was controversy associated with its early roots in the eugenics movement.

Porphyria – a group of disorders of the metabolism of the heme pigment in the blood. Some forms may first manifest during pregnancy.

Position – the placement of an object, body or body part in relationship to any other.

      lithotomy position – a position in which the patient is lying on her back, with her buttocks at the end of the examining table and her hips and knees fully flexed, with the thighs turned outward (frog-legged), usually with her feet supported in stirrups. This is the position most commonly used for gynecologic procedures, including surgical abortion in the first trimester.

Pre-eclampsia – pregnancy-induced high blood pressure. Usually occurs after 20 weeks, but may appear earlier in some circumstances (multiple pregnancy).

Pregnancy – condition of a woman from the time of conceiving an embryo until delivery of the fetus.

      high-risk pregnancy – a pregnancy in which the mother or the fetus or the newborn may be at greater risk of dying or having significant disease before or after delivery. Recognized risk factors are lack of prenatal care, pre-existing maternal disease, poor nutrition, genetic disorders, and unwanted pregnancy.

Pregnant – the state of carrying a developing fetus within the uterus.

Premature – occurring before the expected time.

Prenatal – before birth.

Primigravida – woman who has been pregnant only once.

Primipara – woman who has delivered one child.

Progesterone – a hormone produced in the ovary. Progesterone is necessary for the establishment and maintenance of pregnancy and stimulates the uterine wall to become receptive to the implantation of the embryo.

Progestagen, progestin – a natural or synthetic substance or drug that acts like progesterone.

Pro-Choice – term used to describe those who believe that women should have the choice to decide themselves whether to continue with a pregnancy or to have that pregnancy terminated. 'Pro-choice' implies a belief in the need for legal, safe abortion that is easily accessible financially and geographically to women who seek it.

Pro-Life – term used to describe those who are opposed to the concept of induced abortion and by extension to the provision of legal abortion clinics.

Prophylactic – intended to prevent disease. Also a common slang term for a condom.

Prostaglandins – chemical compounds which occur naturally in the body and are also produced synthetically for use as medications. Naturally occurring prostaglandins are involved in bringing about normal menstruation and normal childbirth – they cause contractions of the myometrium. Synthetic prostaglandins include misoprostol, gemeprost and sulprostone; they are used for medical abortion but also for other purposes in obstetric and gynaecological practice e.g. preventing hemorrhage following normal delivery.

      PGE2 – prostaglandin that stimulates the contraction of the uterus and is available as a vaginal suppository for termination of pregnancy between 12 and 20 weeks of gestation. In a gel form, it may be used to prepare the cervix for induction of labor.

PGF2 alpha – a synthetic preparation that is used to induce abortion or to control postpartum hemmorhage.

Protestantism – the attitudes toward abortion vary widely with the various Protestant denominations. The more liberal Protestant churches like the Church of England, Episcopal, and Quakers, are widely pro-choice, while the more conservative and fundamentalist churches are pro-life. The pro-life movement is strongly associated with fundamentalist Protestant sects.

Pruritic urticarial papules of pregnancy – skin rash in pregnancy. It is red and itchy, occurs around the abdomen and thighs and disappears within two weeks of delivery. It happens almost exclusively in first pregnancies.

Pruritus – persistent itchiness if normal appearing skin.

gravidarum – generalized itchiness occurring during pregnancy, usually during the third trimester. It disappears after delivery.

Psychological effects of induced abortion – This is a subject that has been widely studied and written about in medical journals. Not all studies are of high quality but many are. They also differ in how subjects were recruited, how long they were followed up, what were the outcome measures etc but there are some consistent trends:

1   An overwhelming consensus that voluntary termination of pregnancy performed in societies where it is legal and accepted is only rarely associated with immediate or lasting negative psychological consequences in most women. In some cases positive outcomes such as relief have been expressed.

2   There are some factors associated with negative psychological outcomes: previous psychiatric illness, conflict with religious or cultural beliefs, lack of partner or family support, low self-esteem, and termination later in pregnancy. Some studies have shown that women who have an abortion are more likely to have a psychiatric illness or to self-harm following the abortion than are women with pregnancies proceeding to full-term. However this does not mean that these problems were actually caused by the abortion – in many cases they will be a continuation of problems experienced before the abortion was performed.

3   Partner and/or family support improves outcomes. Age is not a factor, outcomes are similar for younger and older women.

4   Negative outcomes are more likely when the pregnancy has been terminated for reasons of fetal abnormality or maternal health and therefore where the woman has not herself made a positive decision for abortion.

Psychosexual – emotional factors related to sex.

Pubescence – the onset of sexual maturation.

Puerto Rico – Abortion is illegal in Puerto Rico unless it is necessary to preserve the life or health of the woman. The constitutionality of this law has been upheld because it is deemed to provide adequate protection for the health of the woman. The penalty for the person providing the abortion is three years imprisonment; the penalty for any woman soliciting or submitting to an abortion not necessary for her life or health is two to five years imprisonment.

Purulent – consisting of, or containing, pus.

Pus – a fluid substance comprised of dead white blood cells and, often, the causative organism.

Pyrexia – fever.

Q

Quiana

I want to tell my story so that other girls can benefit from it. Last year, when I was fifteen, I started partying and hooking up. We were doing some E at the parties and it made it all so much fun. I never thought that I'd get caught. I know girls who have been doing this since they were thirteen, so how come I was so unlucky? Anyway, there I was at the clinic hearing the doctor tell me that I was pregnant. I tell you I was shocked. I just went home and cried and cried. The doctor told me to think it all over and then come in to see her and talk about starting prenatal care or making arrangements to go for an abortion.

I waited a week. I was hoping it would all go away, but of course, it didn't. I just couldn't let my folks know because my grades are so good that they want me to win a scholarship to college. I'd be the first person from my family to go. We live on a reservation and my family has never had very much. They were so proud of me and I just couldn't let them know that I'd let them down. I told the doctor all this stuff and she was way cool. She even hugged me and she said that I was pretty lucky because in our state, the law doesn't make the clinic notify my parents. I knew I couldn't go ahead and have the baby because it would hurt my family so bad; anyway, I'm just a kid and a baby needs a grown-up parent.

The nurse gave me a bunch of information, including the phone numbers and addresses of all the clinics that would take me. She said that my health coverage wouldn't take care of it and that the charge would be around $400, so I'd have to come up with that. Two of my girlfriends helped me get the money together and one of them went with me on the day that I went to have my abortion. I had a surgical abortion – sort of like a sucking out – because then it would be over and I wouldn't take a chance of having to tell my mom. I went home for an overnight with my girlfriend and she watched out for me.

Someday, when things are right and I'm in a relationship, I want to have lots of babies. Right now, I'm first in my high school class and it looks like my folk's dream will come true. Who knows, maybe I'll even become a doctor.

Q

Queensland – Section 226 of the Criminal Code Act 1899 (Qld) criminalizes abortion, which it describes as 'unlawfully supplying any thing (whether substance or instrument) with the intention of procuring an abortion.' Liability for the practice of abortion in Queensland has traditionally been avoided in the defence in section 282 of the same Act, which allows for 'surgical operations' on the child or mother 'for the preservation of the mother's life if the performance of the operation is reasonable, having regard to the patient's state at the time and all the circumstances of the case.'

A broad interpretation of the section was applied by Justice Maguire in what appears to be the only prosecution made under this section, in the case of 1986 involving Dr Bayliss, who was acquitted. Maguire's interpretation of 'reasonable' has been such as to allow practitioners a degree of flexibility in interpreting the legislation and no further prosecutions have since been brought although abortion remains part of the criminal code.

It would seem that the section 282 defence would not extend to the administration of **mifepristone** (RU 486), as it is clearly not a 'surgical operation.'. In April 2006, after seeking advice from the Solicitor-General, the Premier and the Attorney General issued a joint statement in which the Queensland government took the view that where the Federal TGA has approved use of a drug, prescription of that drug is lawful in Queensland pursuant to the Health (Drugs and Poisons) Regulation 1996 (Qld), and that further amendment to Queensland legislation is not required. Because a prescription is lawful, it is not an unlawful supply, and therefore there is no application of sections 224 or 226 of the Criminal Code Act.

In practice surgical abortion is available in free-standing clinics in large towns throughout Queensland and from certain medical practitioners in smaller towns and rural areas. A small number of first trimester abortions are performed in public and private hospitals. Late abortion usually for fetal abnormality diagnosed after 16 weeks of pregnancy is performed in public and private hospitals which offer antenatal screening for such abnormalities. Medical abortion using **methotrexate** and/or **misoprostol** is available from individual practitioners and some free-standing clinics and mifepristone has recently become available to a limited extent.

Quickening – the feeling of fetal movements by the mother for the first time in a pregnancy. In medieval times it was believed by both Christians and Jews that the soul did not enter the child until the time of quickening (generally about 18-20 weeks in a woman having her first baby and 15-16 weeks in a woman having a second or subsequent baby) therefore abortion was permissible up till that time.

R

Ruth

I'm 41 years old, divorced for the past ten years. I haven't been in any kind of proper relationship since the day my ex-husband walked out on me. I have one son, 20 years old, he lives in another state now and we don't see each other much. It was hard for me taking care of him after his father left and he moved out of home when he was 16. I work for a furniture company, in accounts. I live in rented accommodation and I have to help my sisters keep our mother in a nursing home. We want to care for her decently but it's not cheap.

Last Christmas at the office party I got involved with this man. A real stereotype situation, of course he's one of my bosses and of course he's married. I know about contraceptives, I'm stupid but not that stupid, and we used them. There were only a couple of times then it was over for both of us. Or so I thought. It took me a couple of weeks to realize I'd missed my period. I did a home pregnancy test and it was positive.

There was no way I could tell this man. There was no way I could afford to keep the baby and I was worried it might be abnormal anyway, at my age. Plus, the thought of being a single Mom again just made me feel cold inside. I knew I couldn't cope.

I went interstate. I wanted to have it done with general anesthetic and I went to a clinic in a city where no-one knew me. I couldn't have done it with those pills, at home. I just wanted to be out of it and have it over.

I had an abortion, before, when I was 18. It wasn't exactly legal then but at least a doctor did it. The first time, it didn't worry me, I thought I had my whole life in front of me to have kids, and a friend went with me to the doctor's office. This time I have to say was harder. I just couldn't tell my sisters or anybody else what I'd done. I go to Mass every week but I couldn't talk to the priest and I haven't said what I've done in Confession. The nurses in the clinic were nice but rushed off their feet and no time for any talk. I had to take a cab from the clinic to the bus station and then five hours on the bus home on my own, bleeding quite a bit.

It cost a lot from my savings and I won't be having a vacation for quite a while. I'm sorry I had to have the abortion, I would like to have been a different person with a different life, and kept the baby. But I'm not, and I know I made the right decision for me.

R

Rape – a nonconsensual act of sexual penetration of any body orifice. This is illegal. Rape is usually accomplished by some form of coercion, including physical force, intimidation, deceit, or by impairing the victim's ability to resist, for example by the use of drugs, or by any other means that results in the victim complying against her/his will.

    date rape – when rapes occurs in the context of a social engagement and by a perpetrator known to the victim.

    statutory rape – when sexual intercourse occurs between a minor and an adult. The definitions of minor and adult in this context differ from state to state and adult may be defined to include another minor if that person is a defined number of years older than the victim.

Rates, of abortion – These vary depending on the legal status of abortion and the accessibility of abortion clinics. In the United States about 2% of all women of reproductive age (accepted to be 15-44 years) undergo an abortion each year. This translates into a rate of 17 abortions per 1000 women of reproductive age per year. Another way of describing the abortion rate is the number of abortions per 1000 live births, in the US there are 250 abortions per 1000 live births, that is, one in five pregnancies will have abortion induced. In Australia accurate figures for numbers of induced abortions are not kept but it is estimated that around 80,000-90,000 induced abortions occur each year while total live births are about 250,000, giving a rate of about 1:4 pregnancies terminated by induced abortion. When looked at as numbers of abortions per 1000 women of reproductive age the estimated rates in Australia were 17.9 per 1000 in 1985, rising to 21.9 per 1000 in 1995 and declining somewhat to 19.7 per 1000 in 2003. See also headings under names of individual countries.

Reasons for legal abortion – While details differ from country to country, the following are the main grounds on which abortion is permitted:
1   to save the life of the mother
2   to preserve the physical or mental health of the mother
3   when the pregnancy is the result of rape or incest –
4   when fetal abnormality is likely
5   for compelling socio-economic reasons
6   in a few countries, abortion is available on demand.

RCOG – Royal College of Obstetricians and Gynecologists

Refusal to treat – refusal by a health professional or facility to institute or continue treatment of a patient. Some states grant the right of refusal to treat to specific facilities and health professionals in regard to abortion, in some cases including complications resulting from abortion. These refusals are to be for moral or religious reasons and usually are to be filed in writing.

Regrets, following abortion – see **psychological effects of induced abortion**

Restell, Madame – pseudonym of Ann Lohman, an abortionist who used aggressive advertising and marketing techniques to build a very lucrative abortion business from the early 1830s until 1878, when she committed suicide after being indicted by Anthony

Comstock under the anti-obscenity laws. At the height of her success, she had clinics in New York, Boston and Philadelphia and her publications and mail order business reached many more communities.

Retained products of conception – the medical term used to describe the situation when the abortion process, either medical or surgical, or a natural miscarriage, is incomplete so some of the tissue making up the pregnancy – usually placenta and/or membranes, less commonly part of the fetus – remains inside the uterus. This may be associated with moderate to heavy bleeding and there is the possibility that the tissue may become infected by bacteria migrating from the vagina or bowel. Treatment may include antibiotics and removing the retained material (D&C) under some form of anesthesia in an operating theatre or suitable clinic surroundings. If there is only a small amount of tissue present (which may be confirmed by ultrasound scan) and the woman is not bleeding heavily it may be possible to wait and allow the tissue to be passed naturally or **misoprostol** may be administered to assist this process.

Rhode Island – rated D by **NARAL**. Rhode Island has an unconstitutional and unenforceable ban on abortion as early as 12 weeks. Only physicians are allowed to perform legal abortions in Rhode Island and they are subject to regulations and restrictions that are not applied to physicians in regard to other procedures. A woman may not have an abortion until after she has been informed of the gestational age of the fetus, a description of the abortion procedure to be used and its possible risks, and has signed a state-prepared form that includes a statement of her awareness of the options of foster care and adoption, should she carry her pregnancy to term. A requirement that all married women notify their husbands prior to obtaining an abortion has been found unconstitutional. No physician or other health care personnel can be compelled to participate in abortion services. The person must refuse in writing and give moral or religious grounds as their reason. Rhode Island has an unconstitutional and unenforceable law that no health insurance plan in the state may cover abortion services except in the cases of threat to the woman's life and of pregnancy resulting from rape or incest. It provides that an individual may buy a rider to her policy providing broader abortion coverage. Rhode Island prohibits the use of public funds for abortion except in those cases in which the woman's life is endangered or the pregnancy has resulted from rape or incest. A young woman under 18 years of age must obtain the consent of one parent before she can obtain an abortion. The exceptions are in cases of 'emergency requiring immediate action' or if she is able to obtain a court order allowing her to obtain the abortion. Rhode Island prohibits abortion after viability. It defines viability as a beating heart, electronically-measureable brain waves, movement and development consistent with extra-uterine life with access to usual medical care. The only exception is to preserve the life of the woman. Rhode Island requires that any health insurance plan that covers prescription drugs provide the same coverage for contraception.

Risks, of abortion – see Safety

Rockefeller Foundation – major donor to abortion reform in the 1970s.

Roe, Jane – pseudonym of Norma McCorvey, who challenged the Texas anti-abortion laws, resulting in the landmark Roe vs Wade decision of the US Supreme Court.

Roe vs. Wade – landmark US Supreme Court decision of 1973 that legalized abortion in the US. In 1970, Jane Roe (a pseudonym to protect the identity of Norma McCorvey, the woman involved) instituted action against Henry Wade, the district attorney of Dallas

County, TX, to prevent him enforcing the state anti-abortion law on the grounds that the law was unconstitutional. The law dated from the 1850s (see History of abortion in the US) and had been interpreted to prohibit abortion at any stage except as advised by a doctor in order to save the life of the woman. The decision in the case was rendered in January 1973 in Jane Roe's favor. The law, and by extension, all similar state laws (in at least 41 states and the District of Columbia) was found to be unconstitutional. It was the opinion of the Court that in abortion policy there was a conflict of a number of separately legitimate social concerns. These were 1) the right of the individual to privacy in intimate matters 2) the right of the state to protect maternal health and 3) the right of the state to protect developing life. In adjudicating the prioritization of these rights, the Court viewed pregnancy as separated into its three trimesters. It ruled that during the first trimester of pregnancy, the woman's right to privacy took precedence over the other rights, basically granting to women the legal right to abortion on demand during the first trimester. In the second trimester, the right of the state to regulate and protect maternal health takes precedence. This means that the state can still not deny the woman an abortion, but can insist upon more control over the standards of medical procedures. In the third trimester, the state's 'legitimate interest in potential life' overrides the woman's right to determine her own decision without government intervention. The state may proscribe abortion except when necessary to preserve the life or health of the mother. In this decision, the Court majority defined viability as that point at which a fetus can survive outside the womb, with or without artificial aids, and implicitly denied that human life existed in a legally meaningful form prior to viability. The Justices found that the right of privacy, whether founded in the Fourteenth Amendment's explication of personal liberty and restrictions on State action, or in the Ninth Amendment' reservation of rights to the people, is broad enough to encompass a woman's decision whether or not to terminate her pregnancy. The majority decision was written by Justice Blackmun, who also wrote of the safety of first trimester abortion compared with childbirth. He based this concept on the *amicus curiae* brief filed by the **American College of Obstetricians and Gynecologists** in the case of Doe vs Bolton. In this brief, early abortion was estimated to be twenty-three times safer than childbirth at full term.

Romalis, Garson – Vancouver, BC doctor who was shot and wounded on 8 November 1994 by an anti-abortion activist.

Rothman, Lorraine – inventor, together with Carol Downer, of the **Del-M** device.

Roussel Uclaf – French pharmaceutical company (previously part of the German Hoechst group) which conducted much of the research leading to the development of the drug RU 486 (RU=Roussel Uclaf) during the early 1980s

Royal College of Obstetricians and Gynaecologists – United Kingdom specialist body, has produced comprehensive guidelines for the practice of abortion by doctors including legal and ethical concerns and the keeping of accurate records. Guidelines include evidence-based medical recommendations for safe abortion practice.

RU-486 – laboratory name of mifepristone, first synthesized by the company Roussel Uclaf .

Rubella – a communicable viral disease, also called German measles, usually mild and of short duration, but capable of causing severe fetal deformities when a mother has rubella in the first trimester of pregnancy. Today, most women are immunized against rubella before they become pregnant as part of the system of childhood immunizations.

Rudolph, Eric – convicted of the 1998 murder of Robert Sanderson, an off-duty police officer who was guarding an abortion clinic. Rudolph received a life sentence. He was also charged for the bombing at the Atlanta Olympics.

S

Sadie

All the time I was growing up, I thought it would be so great to be a Mom. I was something of a misfit: old parents, no brothers or sisters and only really old relatives. I'd watch my friends with their family fun and be really jealous. I got pregnant in high school and had to quit school. My folks were still alive then and they wouldn't have heard of any other solution: I was 'in trouble' and that's what girls did then, at least in our town. The boy didn't know me no more at all and in those days you just didn't take a guy to court.

After little Billy was born, we stayed with my folks, but when he was nine months old, my mother died. She was old and she had a bad heart anyway. So it was me and Dad and little Bill. Dad had a little pension from working on the railroads and I worked at the local greasy spoon. We got by. Then when Billy was three, my dad died, too, and things got real hard. The county took our house for taxes and Billy and I had to move in to a rooming house. The owner liked kids so for a while she watched him when I worked. I had to work a lot to make ends meet even without having much. Then I got the flu one fall and couldn't work for a week. I got behind on the rent and she threw us out.
It was lucky that Billy was five by then and I could sign him up for kindergarten and the after-school program at the school. I was lucky we had that. Not all places even had kindergarten. Anyway, I had two jobs then – one at the lunch counter and on at Ames. The Ames job gave me a discount on stuff so I could get Billy some clothes for school. Me, I got my clothes from Good Will. I was always tired and Billy and I were living in a friend's apartment. We had to share a bed and sometimes he still wet the bed. It was hard, but at least we were together.

One guy who hung out at the restaurant started sweet talking me and it was good to feel like a woman for a little while each day. He wasn't much to look at but he was nice to me. Nobody'd looked at me since that guy in high school. Anyway, one thing led to another, although even that wasn't easy. He had a little apartment but his landlady was a nosy bodkins and we had to sneak around. Before I knew it, I was pregnant again. When I told him, he went ballistic and said that I wasn't no virgin; I should take care of myself. Two days later, he cleared out and left no forwarding address (though I don't know if the landlady would give it to me anyway).

So now here I was with a bun in the oven and no one to help out. For a couple of weeks, I tried to pretend that it wasn't true, but then common sense took hold and I knew something had to be done. I went to the welfare office, waited on line for an hour and then got to talk to a social worker. She told me I could go to Planned Parenthood and gave me their address and phone number. She said I could get food stamps, too, and some money to help take care of Billy. Don't know why I never went there before.

So, I went to Planned Parenthood and they fixed me up. They told me about a pill that I can take to keep from getting pregnant, if I want to. And my stuff is free with them. How could I get to be in the middle of my twenties and not know about these things?

Well, now I do. I felt bad about getting rid of a baby, but it was better than the life I could give him.

S

Safety, of abortion – Problems at the time of a legal abortion or soon afterwards are uncommon. The risk of death overall from an abortion performed legally in a hospital or clinic, in the US, Europe, UK or Australia, is about one woman in 100,000. This can be compared with the risk of dying if a pregnancy proceeds to full term, which is 10-12 women per 100,000 pregnant women (the maternal mortality rate) in these countries. The risk of excessive bleeding (hemorrhage) requiring blood transfusion is around one in every 500-1000 abortions before 12 weeks and somewhat greater in later abortions. Damage to the cervix may occur in up to ten surgical abortions in 1,000 (see also **cervical incompetence, cervical dilatation**). Perforation of the uterus at the time of induced surgical abortion up to 12 weeks of pregnancy occurs in about four per 1000 abortions; rupture of the uterus happens in less than one in 1000 medical abortions done after 12 weeks and is virtually unknown before 12 weeks.. Approximately 5% of surgical abortions are complicated by infection requiring antibiotic treatment.

Salpingitis – infection and inflammation of the fallopian tubes usually as part of a general pelvic inflammatory disease.

Salvi, John – murdered Leann Nichols and Shannon Lowry in 1994 attack on two abortion clinics in Boston, MA. He was found to be insane and committed suicide while in jail.

Sanderson, Robert – Birmingham, AL policeman who was murdered by Eric Rudolph in 1998. Sanderson was off-duty and guarding an abortion clinic at the time of the shooting.

Sanger, Margaret – 1883 – 1966. American pioneer of birth control (she invented the term). Born in Corning, New York, she became a nurse and worked on New York City's Lower East Side where she saw firsthand the effects of too many pregnancies on women and their families, and the practice of illegal abortion. Traveled to Europe in search of information on methods of family limitation, on her return to the US in mid-1914 published a monthly news sheet, *The Woman Rebel*, and a pamphlet, *Family Limitations*. These attracted the attention of **Comstock** and were barred from the mails. Thus began a life of advocacy of contraception as a right for women and the dissemination of birth control information, a struggle that included detention in the workhouse and frequent arrests and charges in court. In 1916 Sanger opened a birth control clinic in Brooklyn that immediately attracted hundreds of women seeking advice – and the attention of the vice squad. Again imprisoned, while there the first issue of her broadsheet *Birth Control Review* appeared – the journal was to appear regularly until 1940. On her release she traveled constantly lecturing – her main opposition came from the hierarchy of the Catholic church. In November 1921 the first American National Birth Control Conference launched the American Birth Control League with Margaret Sanger as president. In 1923 she founded her Clinical Research Bureau, in 1929 the National Committee on Federal Legislation for Birth Control, which gradually attracted support for the idea of birth control from the medical profession (and financial support from her second husband, a wealthy oil magnate.) She gained an international reputation, organizing the Sixth International Conference on Birth Control in New York in 1925 and the World Population Conference in Geneva in 1927. In 1929 police carried out a raid on the Clinical Research Bureau in which patient files were illegally seized and names made public. The case generated enormous publicity for the work of the Bureau and for Margaret Sanger's work generally. Birth control clinics began to appear all across the US although there continued to be sporadic police raids up until the Second World War. In 1948 Margaret Sanger helped form the **International Planned Parenthood Federation** and later became the IPPF's President Emeritus.

Sedation – Some clinics and hospitals use drugs given intravenously (into a vein) just before a surgical abortion procedure. When drugs are used which alter consciousness by making the woman significantly drowsy this is called 'conscious sedation'. The aim of this is to make the woman feel more relaxed and experience minimal pain from the procedure. The use of conscious sedation requires closer monitoring of the patient during the time that consciousness is altered

Side-effects, of drugs – unlooked-for effects of drugs, in addition to the desired therapeutic effects. Side-effects may be harmful or beneficial.

Short, Hugh – doctor in Ancaster, Ontario who was shot while eating his breakfast on Nov. 10, 1995. James Kopp, who was convicted of killing Dr. Barnett Slepian, has been charged with Dr. Short's assault.

Slepian, Barnett – Amherst, NY obstetrician/gynecologist who was murdered by James Kopp in Oct. 1998. Dr. Slepian was in the kitchen of his home, with his family present, and Kopp shot him through the window, using a high-powered assault rifle.

South Australia – Abortion can be performed in South Australia if the pregnancy is under 28 weeks and 'the continuation of the pregnancy involves greater risk to a woman's life or there is a risk of injury to physical or mental health, taking into account her actual or reasonably foreseeable environment' or there are serious physical or mental abnormalities in the fetus.

There is a two months residency requirement in South Australia; two doctors must agree that the abortion is indicated and it must be carried out in a 'prescribed' clinic or hospital.

South Carolina – rated F by **NARAL**. South Carolina has an unconstitutional and unenforceable ban on abortion as early as twelve weeks. There is a post-viability restriction prohibiting any abortion after 24 weeks unless physicians certify that it is necessary to preserve the woman's life or health. Only physicians are allowed to perform legal abortions and they are subject to regulations and restrictions not applied to other physicians performing other procedures. State employees are prohibited from counseling or referring women for abortion; also, funds available under the South Carolina Birth Defects Program may not be used to counsel or refer for abortion. A woman may not have an abortion until after she is counseled by a health professional about the procedure to be done and is informed of the gestational age of the fetus. She must also be given state-prepared materials to read and may not have the abortion until one hour after reading these materials. A married woman who lives with her husband may not obtain a third-trimester abortion without her husband's consent; this provision has been found unconstitutional. No healthcare worker may be required to participate in abortion services after submitting their refusal in writing. However, in emergency circumstances, no hospital may refuse admittance. State funds may not be used for abortion except to preserve the life of the woman or in cases where the pregnancy is the result of rape or incest. A minor woman under age 17, who has never been married or emancipated, must obtain the witnessed signed consent of one parent or grandparent before she may obtain an abortion. This requirement may be waived if the pregnancy is the result of incest or if the minor obtains a judicial order. South Carolina law provides that victims of sexual assault have access to emergency contraception through emergency rooms.

South Dakota – rated F by **NARAL**. South Dakota has enacted a ban on abortion at any stage of gestation unless the abortion is necessary to preserve the woman's life. This ban went into effect 1 July, 2006 and is unconstitutional and unenforceable according to existing federal law. A challenge to this SD law was included on the ballot in South Dakota for the November, 2006 Congressional elections: on 7 November, the voters of SD rejected the abortion ban that had been passed by their legislature. Exit polls indicated that the voters felt that the ban did not provide adequate protections for the woman in cases of rape or incest. In the South Dakota state code there is language expressing the state's opposition to abortion and intent to restrict reproductive choice to the greatest extent possible. South Dakota only allows physicians to perform legal abortions and imposes restrictions and regulations on these physicians that are not imposed on other physicians for other procedures. South Dakota requires pre-abortion counseling in two phases: at least 24 hours prior to having an abortion, a woman must receive state-prepared written materials and at least two hours prior to having an abortion, she must be told by the physician the name of the physician who will perform the procedure, that abortion ends the life of a human being with whom she has a relationship and that the rights attendant upon this relationship under law will end with the abortion. She must also be told the gestational age of the fetus and the risks of the procedure. There is currently an injunction against this counseling requirement because it violated the First Amendment rights of the physician; this injunction is currently being appealed in the US Court of Appeals. No healthcare worker, social worker, medical facility or other person can be required to participate in abortion services and no pharmacist can be required to fill any prescription that could be used to cause abortion. South Dakota prohibits the use of public funds for abortion unless the procedure is necessary to preserve the woman's life. A minor woman under 18 may not obtain an abortion until at least 48 hours after one parent is notified in writing. This may be waived only for a certified medical emergency or by court order.

Spain – Abortion is legal and widely available. The law provides for abortion to be done for cases of rape or incest, for fetal abnormality and in cases where the life or health of the mother are at risk – 97% of abortions come into the latter category. About 16% of pregnancies to Spanish residents end in abortion; Spain is also increasingly a destination for abortion 'tourists' – women who find accessing abortion in their own countries difficult. In particular women from Ireland and Malta travel to Spain for abortion.

State lines, crossing over for abortion

Australia – there is no legislation in Australia forbidding the crossing of state borders for the purpose of procuring an abortion. It is known (from Medicare data) that approximately 2,500. Queensland women travel interstate each year in order to undergo abortion and that several hundred women annually travel to Victoria from other states in order to obtain late abortions.

US – there is no legislation forbidding the crossing of borders for the purpose of obtaining an abortion. If the woman is eligible for public medical funding (Medicaid), her eligibility for a publicly funded abortion would be determined by the laws of the states involved.

Sterilization – surgical operation performed as a permanent method of contraception

      female – clips or rings are placed on the Fallopian tubes or a part or all of each tube is removed, known as tubal ligation

      male – vasectomy – the vas, the tube which carries sperm from the testis to the outside world is occluded on each side with a permanent tie

Stopes, Marie – 1880 – 1958. born in Edinburgh, Scotland. She obtained a Doctor of Science in 1905. During World War I, she wrote and published *Married Life*, in which she argued that marriage should be an equal partnership between a man and a woman. The book was a success in Britain and banned in the USA. In 1918, she wrote a concise guide to birth control called *Wise Parenthood*. In 1921, she founded the Society for Constructive Birth Control and opened the first family planning clinic in the United Kingdom. This, the Mothers' Clinic is still operating in Central London. She continued to open more clinics and was instrumental in the formation of the National Birth Control Council. Stopes was also a prominent eugenics activist.

Storer, Horatio R. – former Harvard Professor of Obstetrics and Gynecology. In 1868. with his colleague, lawyer Franklin Fiske Heard, published the most careful and systematic calculation of mid-century American abortion rates yet done. They were assisted by Dr. Elisha Harris, who was Registrar of Vital Statistics in New York City. They found that reported early abortions had a ratio of 1 to 4.04 living births in New York City. They suggested that from their research, these figures were likely true for most other US localities. Storer was an anti-abortion activist and headed the AMA campaign against abortion from its inception in 1850.

Suction curettage – the use of a firm plastic cannula attached to a suction pump for the purpose of emptying the cavity of the uterus (womb) during the process of surgical abortion up to 14 weeks of pregnancy. The cannula is a wide bore tube open at both ends. One end is joined by tubing to the suction pump, the other has a sharp edge which is used to curette (scrape) the inside walls of the uterus to ensure that all pregnancy tissue is removed. Also known as **vacuum aspiration.**

Sulprostone – synthetic prostaglandin used for medical abortion in 1980s, no longer widely used

Sunnen Foundation – major donor to abortion reform in the 1970s.

Surgical abortion – abortion performed using a suction curette or instruments to extract the products of conception from the uterus and curette (scrape) the walls of the cavity of the uterus. Some form of dilatation of the cervical canal is needed before surgical extraction of the pregnancy can be performed – this may be with a drug such as misoprostol, devices such as laminaria tents or graded surgical dilators which are passed through the canal by the operator. Surgical abortion procedures are painful and analgesia and/or anesthesia should be provided. Surgical abortion can be safely performed up to 14 weeks of pregnancy in a clinic or hospital but must be performed by a trained and experienced health professional, usually a physician in those countries where abortion is legal. After 14 weeks abortion can safely be performed surgically, by dilating the cervix, removing the fetus and placenta and curetting the uterus (D&E) but the best results are obtained by physicians specializing in these techniques as the risks of bleeding (hemorrhage) and damage to both the cervix and to adjacent tissues are greater than with abortion done in early pregnancy. In general for surgical abortion techniques using suction curettage have replaced the use of steel instruments as complication rates are less.

Sussman, Frank – lawyer who argued pro-choice stance in Webster v. Reproductive Health Services. Strong advocate of the right to privacy in reproductive issues.

Sweden – abortion legal since 1975. Up to 18 weeks of pregnancy the decision regarding abortion is the woman's own; counseling is offered but is not mandatory. After 18 weeks an application must be made to the National Board of Health and Welfare; counseling is compulsory and the application must be made jointly by a gynecologist and the social worker/counselor. Around 40,000 abortions per year are performed in Sweden. Both surgical and medical methods are widely available. Medical abortion may take place entirely in a clinic or hospital or the woman may be administered mifepristone in the clinic and given misoprostol for self-administration at home.

T

Tammy

I grew up in a little town where everyone knew everyone else. This was mostly good, but when I was in my last year of high school, I got pregnant. It was so stupid, really; I wasn't going with anyone or anything like that. It was just a warm spring night and too much beer.

When I missed my period, I went to the Planned Parenthood clinic in the little city twenty miles away and they told me that I was pregnant. The counselor sat down with me right away and told me all the options open to me. In my state, if you are under eighteen, your parents have to consent to an abortion, but I had just turned eighteen, so at least I didn't have that to face. The only clinic that does abortions is seventy-five miles away and I'd have to come up with about $400. She also told me that I could consider adoption and gave me the names and phone numbers of several agencies that help girls who want their babies to be adopted. Or, I could keep the baby.

At first, I just wanted to have the abortion and not have to face telling my folks. I kept trying to call the number for the clinic, but I'd put the receiver down as soon as it started to ring. I called the counselor and went back in to talk with her some more. Talking with her, I realized that even though I'm not a real churchy Catholic, still I just couldn't bring myself to have an abortion. I really am afraid that it is a mortal sin.

So, I faced the scene of telling my mother and father. It went better than I ever dreamed it would and they have been very supportive. I looked into all the agencies that handle adoptions but I decided to wait until the end to decide. I'm glad I did because there is no way I could have given my Meredith away. Mom and Pop have been really good to me. I'm taking classes at the community college and Mom takes care of Meredith when I have to be away. I got Medicaid for Meredith and that takes care of all her check-ups and stuff. I finally told the guy who is Meredith's father and he wants to be part of her life, so he visits often and he gives me money to help with her needs.

T

Tasmania – has abortion incorporated into the criminal code similarly to Victoria but there has been no testing in case law. Sections 134 and 135 of the Criminal Code cover abortion which is performed in free-standing clinics.

Teratogen – a substance that damages or has the potential to damage an embryo or fetus, causing the infant to be born with abnormalities if the pregnancy continues. Drugs used for medical abortion including **methotrexate** and **misoprostol** can act as teratogens if the abortion is unsuccessful and the pregnancy proceeds. Many drugs used for other purposes like the antibiotics of the tetracycline group and the anti-acne drug isotretinoin are teratogens; taking such drugs in early pregnancy may be an indication for an induced abortion.

Term – a definite time period.

      full-term – pregnancy of 36 – 42 weeks duration.

Termination of pregnancy – deliberately ending a pregnancy so that it does not progress to birth.

Termination Review Committee – a committee that makes decisions or recommendations as to the ethical and legal advisability of proceeding on specific requests for late term abortion. These committees are comprised of clinicians, including the attending physician and a pediatrician, and may include hospital or clinic administrative officers. Consultation may be requested by the committee with lawyers or ethicists. Such a scheme exists in the state of **Victoria**, Australia.

Tennessee – rated D+ by **NARAL**. Tennessee has an unconstitutional and unenforceable ban on abortion as early as twelve weeks. No post-viability abortion may be done unless it is necessary to preserve the life or health of the woman; the certificate of necessity must be filed with the attorney general prior to performing the abortion. Tennessee requires that written consent be obtained from a woman prior to an abortion; other counseling and delay requirements have been found unconstitutional under the Tennessee State Constitution. Only physicians are allowed to perform legal abortions in Tennessee and these physicians are subject to regulations and restrictions not placed on other physicians doing other procedures. No physician or hospital may be required to participate in abortion services. Also, private medical facilities and physicians and the employees of either may refuse to provide contraception or contraceptive information if the refusal is based on religion or conscience. Tennessee prohibits the use of public funds for abortion unless it is necessary to preserve the life of the woman or the pregnancy is the result of rape or incest. A minor woman under 18 may not obtain an abortion until the physician obtains the signed written consent of one parent. This may be waived if there is a criminal charge of incest against a parent or if the physician certifies that a medical emergency exists. It may also be waived by court order. These restrictions have also been interpreted to apply to mifepristone.

Testis – one of two paired glands in the male that produce sperm and hormones (mostly testosterone.)

Testosterone – the most potent of the naturally produced male hormones.

Tetracycline – common antibiotic that can cause abnormalities of the fetal bones and developing teeth if taken by the woman during pregnancy.

Texas – rated F by **NARAL**. Texas prohibits third-trimester abortion unless it is necessary to preserve the woman's life or prevent brain damage or paralysis or if the fetus has a severe and irreversible abnormality. A woman may not obtain an abortion until at least 24 hours after the physician informs her of the gestational age of the fetus and the risks of the procedure, as well as those of carrying the pregnancy to term. She must also receive a state-mandated lecture from the physician or his agent, reading from state-prepared materials. These materials are available on the State of Texas Department of Health website. Only physicians are allowed to perform legal abortions in Texas and they are subject to regulations and restrictions not imposed on other doctors performing other procedures. Any healthcare worker or facility may refuse to participate in abortion services. In an emergency situation, no hospital may refuse admittance to the patient. Texas prohibits the use of public funds for abortion unless it is necessary to preserve the life of the woman or if the pregnancy is the result of rape or incest. A minor woman under 18, who is not married or emancipated, must obtain the consent of one parent at least 48 hours prior to having an abortion. This may be waived only in case of medical emergency or by judicial order.

Thalassemia – group of hereditary disorders that are characterized by defects in hemoglobin production and sometimes, anemia.

Therapeutic exception – allows legal abortion when it is deemed medically necessary to preserve the life or health of the woman. First seen in the New York State criminal code of 1828.

Therapeutic Goods Administration – Federal body in Australia charged with assessing the safety and efficacy of drugs prior to licensing in Australia. Has a similar role to the **FDA** in the United States

Thrombophlebitis – inflammation of a vein occurring in association with the formation of a clot in the vein.

Thyroiditis – inflammation of the thyroid.

Thyrotoxicosis – an excess of thyroid hormone leading to response of body organs, with increased heart rate, increased body temperature, tremors, diarrhea. Can be life-threatening if metabolic control is not achieved (then referred to as thyroid storm) and in pregnancy, can threaten the pregnancy.

Timing, of abortions – In the United States (year 2000 figures) 58% of abortions are performed before 8 weeks of pregnancy and 88% before 13 weeks. Recommended abortion methods for different periods of gestation (weeks of pregnancy) are as follows:
4–9 weeks – medical abortion using mifepristone or methotrexate followed by misoprostol
7–14 weeks – surgical abortion using suction curettage, under general or local anesthesia
12–20+ weeks – medical abortion using prostaglandins (misoprostol or gemeprost) +/- mifepristone or surgical dilatation and evacuation of the uterus by specialist practitioners.

Transdermal – applied on or entering through the skin. Also called transcutaneous. Examples are the contraceptive patch and the hormone replacement patch.

Trimester – a period of three months. Traditionally pregnancy has been divided into three trimesters each of approximately 12-13 weeks. Up to the end of the first trimester approximately, surgical abortion is considered safe to perform using suction curettage.

Beyond this time abortion is induced by medical means or by dilation and evacuation or dilation and extraction, because the fetus, placenta and membranes are too large to remove by suction alone. The concept of trimesters was incorporated into the Roe v. Wade decision of 1973 that legalized abortion in the United States. Induced abortion in the first trimester was considered to be a private matter between the woman and her doctor. In fact pregnancy is a continuous process with no sharp divisions into different phases and the concept of trimesters in practice is somewhat artificial. See **timing of abortion.**

> **first trimester** – in pregnancy, the period from the time of fertilization through 14 weeks.
> **second trimester** – the 15th – 28th weeks of pregnancy.
> **third trimester** – the 29th – 42nd weeks of pregnancy.

Trophoblast – tissue that is initially part of the developing embryo and which later differentiates into the placenta

Trosch, David C – a Catholic priest in Mobile, Al who has preached and written materials advocating violence to stop abortion. He runs a website advocating the same. He was a friend and supporter of Paul Hill. Trosch has been removed from his Mobile, AL parish because of his militant anti-abortion activities, which have not been condoned by the Catholic church in the US

U

Ursula

I was born in 1943, conceived during two days leave my father had from the Army during World War II. I never knew him as he was killed two weeks later. My mother managed bringing up three of us on her own after that. She had a government widow's pension but it wasn't easy for her.

From when I was 16 my boyfriend was Colin. We lived in the same part of town and went to school together. When we left school, Colin began as an apprentice in cabinet making and I did a secretarial course. We didn't earn much and we lived at home. Sex before marriage was frowned upon then and very harsh things were said about girls who were rumored to 'go all the way.' When Colin and I were both 19, we got secretly engaged and we began to have sex. It was difficult to find a place for this, he would have to borrow his Dad's car and we would go to the drive-in or out of town. We used condoms for contraception and for about six months that worked okay. Then I missed my periods. I went to a doctor in the next town who did a test – it took a week to get the results then and in that time I was getting sick, throwing up and more and more certain I was pregnant. Colin and I talked it over, he was willing to get married but we had no money saved and we could not live on his single wage if I had to stop work and look after a baby. Also, my mother would be very shocked to know that I was not a virgin. She expected me to go to Church every Sunday like she did. So when I went back to the doctor who told me I was pregnant, I told him I could not have the baby.

He did not seem surprised but gave me the name of a nurse who did abortions – he would not write it down and said I was never to tell anyone he had done this. I rang the number he gave me and I was told to bring £10 and some pads with me to a certain address two days later. I had to come on my own and tell no-one where I was going. It was in this woman's house. I had to lie on the bed in the back room and have a syringe put in my vagina and into my cervix. She squirted salt solution inside me. It was agony, I thought I would die from the pain and shock of it. I had to stay there a while and then the pain wore off a bit. I began to bleed, and she told me the bleeding would turn into a heavy period and I would pass clots but that the baby was very small and I wouldn't see it come out. If I didn't bleed I should come back and she would do it again and wouldn't want to be paid a second time.

I went home and next day got terrible period cramps and started to bleed. The bleeding and pain got worse and worse, I couldn't go to work and my mother got increasingly worried about me. Then I got a fever and she called our own doctor who was a very nice woman who took one look at me, sent my mother out of the room and said Ursula, I know what's happened and I won't tell your mother but you need to come into the hospital. I had peritonitis. I had antibiotic injections for three weeks and an operation to drain the pus from around my tubes but I did get better. If my mother knew what had caused the peritonitis she never ever said so to me. Colin wasn't allowed in to see me in the hospital and he was terribly worried. It took two months for my convalescence and I lost my job as a result.

After that we were too afraid to have sex but we saved up as much as we could and when we were 24 we were married. By then the pill was available and anyway I was a married woman. I took it for two years then stopped – to have a family, I thought. Eighteen months later I still wasn't pregnant and I had X-rays that showed that my tubes were blocked by the infection I'd had after the abortion. This caused us both a lot of heartache and for a long time I felt guilty about what I'd done. We put our names on the adoption list and when we were in our early thirties we were rewarded by adopting our two sons – Simon who is perfectly normal and Ned who has Down syndrome. In the end our family has worked out for us but I am still angry at the hypocrisy of the society I grew up in. I have supported all the campaigns to have safe abortion in Australia and sex education in schools as I wouldn't want other young women growing up to go through what I did.

U

Ultrasonography – visualization of internal body structures by bouncing high-frequency sound waves off the body tissues and converting the echoes into a pictorial display.

    prenatal – ultrasound done through the abdomen to visualize the pelvic contents, used to date pregnancy and to assess the well-being of the fetus.

    transvaginal -technique utilizing a probe placed within the vagina to examine the uterus, ovaries and tubes.

Ultrasound – commonly used term for process of diagnostic ultrasonography and for the image produced.

Unborn Victims of Violence Act – is a US law passed in 2004 that defines a violent attack against a pregnant woman as two distinct crimes: one against the woman and one against her unborn child. The law applies only to those crimes committed on Federal property, against Federal officials or employees, and by members of the military. This law has been interpreted by some as a step toward granting legal personhood to fetuses, although the law contains a specific exception for abortion.\

United Kingdom – abortion available as per the 1967 **Abortion Act**. In England and Wales (approximately 175,000 abortions annually) around 78% of all abortions are performed on the NHS; 22% are outsourced to bodies such as **bpas**. In Scotland 98% of abortions are performed on the NHS (around 11,000 procedures per year.) Approximately 1500 abortions are performed each year in **Northern Ireland**.

Ureter – long (25 -30 cm or about 10 -12 inches) slender, muscular tube leading from the kidney to the bladder.

Urethra – canal from the bladder to the exterior of the body.

Urethritis – inflammation of the urethra, commonly causing burning while urinating.

    Chlamydial – sexually transmitted disease, caused by *Chlamydia trachomatis*.

    Gonococcal – sexually transmitted disease, caused by *Neisseria gonorrhea*.

    non-gonococcal – sexually transmitted disease caused by a variety of organisms, but most commonly, Chlamydia.

Urinary urgency – a strong urge to urinate.

Urinate – to void or pass urine.

Urine – fluid excreted by the kidneys, stored in the bladder and voided through the urethra. It is normally sterile, and is composed of 96% water and 4% waste material from the bodily processes.

Utah – rated F by **NARAL**. Utah has an unconstitutional and unenforceable ban on abortion throughout pregnancy. It also specifically bans all abortions after 20 weeks unless necessary to preserve the woman's life or health or in cases of severe fetal defects; this has been found unconstitutional because it effectively defines viability and by doing so violates Supreme Court precedent. Utah has expressed its opposition to abortion and its determination to restrict reproductive choice in its state code. A woman may not obtain an abortion until at least 24 hours after a healthcare worker tells her in person of the risks of the proposed procedure to her and how it will effect the fetus, a description of the fetus at the particular gestational age, medical risks of carrying the pregnancy to term, and a discussion of all alternatives to abortion. In addition, she must receive a state mandated lecture, using state-prepared materials, and view a state-prepared video at least 24 hours prior to having an abortion. Utah has an unconstitutional and unenforceable requirement that the husband of any married woman be notified prior to her having an abortion. Only physicians are allowed to perform abortions in Utah and they are subject to regulations and restrictions not imposed on other physicians performing other procedures. Any physician, hospital or hospital employee may refuse on moral or religious grounds to participate in abortion. Utah prohibits public funding of abortion except to preserve the life and health of the woman or if there is a severe fetal defect or if the pregnancy is the result of rape or incest. A minor under 18 may not obtain an abortion until at least 24 hours after the physician notifies one of her parents and obtains written informed consent from one parent. This requirement may be waived only in cases of medical emergency where the minor's life is endangered or in regard to a parent who has abused or sexually abused the minor and there is no other parent. The abuse must be reported. The requirement may also be waived by judicial order.

Uterine – relating to the uterus

Uterine cancer – tumor developing in the lining of the uterus (endometrium) and spreading into the muscular wall (myometrium) of the uterus and down to the cervix. Uterine cancer is associated with diabetes, obesity, polycystic ovarian syndrome (PCOS) and is more common in women who have few or no pregnancies but it has not been shown to be associated in any way with abortion.

Uterine perforation – a risk of surgical abortion, especially in illicit circumstances. The muscular wall of the uterus is pierced by an instrument.

Uterine sound – a slender, tapered instrument used to gauge the depth of the uterus. Sometimes used by illegal abortionists to produce abortion.

Uterus – womb. Organ lined by **endometrium** which is shed each month as periods if a woman has not conceived in that menstrual cycle. If conception has occurred the fertilized ovum (egg) settles into the endometrium and develops into fetus, placenta and membranes if the pregnancy continues

Uterus, cancer of – tumor developing in the endometrium and spreading into the muscular wall (myometrium) of the uterus and down to the cervix. Uterine cancer is associated with diabetes, obesity, polycystic ovarian syndrome (PCOS) and is more common in women who have few or no pregnancies but it has not been shown to be associated in any way with abortion

V

Virginia

I was the ugly duckling, the girl who stood at the back of the room and watched as the other girls flirted and were picked out by the young men at the college mixers. Books were my solace and my true companions and, of course, I did very well, academically. I was fortunate – in my day, women didn't go to MIT and get a graduate degree in physics, but I did. And I loved my work. I stayed in academia and made teaching and research my life.

Long after I'd given up any thoughts of romance, Dennis appeared in my life. He came to the university on a post-doctoral fellowship and we met at a lecture. He wasn't in physics, so I wondered why he was spending time chatting with me. I could advance his knowledge and his career not one jot. And when he asked me to have dinner with him, I thought something must be gone wrong with my hearing. But dinner we did have, not once, but many dinners, and lunches, and eventually, breakfasts. Imagine a thirty-eight year old virgin! He said that I was beautiful. And after six months, he asked me to marry him.

It was a beautiful wedding, simple and full of our love. We were very happy and settled into a most harmonious domestic routine. We never really thought about children. We were both so absorbed in our work and each other that we needed nothing else to complete us. I don't know why we assumed that I wouldn't get pregnant, but I guess we did. For five years, we got away with our terrible innocence, but when I was forty-four, I became pregnant.

The guilt was crushing. That we could be so careless and inconsiderate of one another! There was really very little to discuss. We really did not want to be reluctant elderly parents and we could not see ourselves adequately parenting a child… and what if the child turned out to be defective in some way? It was unconscionable. I went to England and had an early surgical abortion and Dennis almost immediately had a vasectomy.

No, we've never looked back. Of course, we are retired now and sometimes I wonder if a child would be a comfort to us, but there is no point in pursuing that line of thought. We are still completely devoted to one another and there is really no room in our lives for anyone else.

V

Vacuum aspiration – see suction curettage

Vagina – the muscular canal leading from the cervix to the exterior (vulva) of the woman.

Vaginal – relating to the vagina.

Vaginismus – painful spasms of the vagina preventing vaginal examination or sexual intercourse.

Vaginitis – inflammation of the vagina.

Vaginodynia – pain in the vagina.

Vaginosis – disease of the vagina.

       bacterial – infection with bacteria, usually causing a grayish white discharge that causes the woman to feel wet.

Valproic acid – commonly used anticonvulsant medication that can cause birth defects, such as spina bifida, when the mother uses it during the first **trimester**.

Vasectomy – see sterilization, male

Venereal – relating to sexual contact, e.g. venereal disease is sexually transmitted disease.

Ventouse – vacuum extractor to aid in childbirth instead of forceps.

Vermont – rated A by **NARAL**. Legislature is pro-choice. Vermont has not repealed its pre-Roe ban on abortion. Vermont's state constitution provides greater protection for a woman's right to choose than does the US Constitution. Vermont law requires all health insurance plans that cover prescription drugs to also cover contraception. Low income women who qualify for medical assistance under the state programs have access to abortion.

Viable – being able to sustain life.

Victoria (Australian State) – The Crimes Act 1958 (Vic) continues to maintain abortion within the criminal code, following on the legislation enacted in the Offences Against the Person Act of 1861. The crime of administering a drug or using any instrument to procure an abortion (including by a woman herself) is set out in section 65, and that of unlawful supply of such drug or instrument is in section 66.

       The Menhennitt decision in the Davidson case of 1969 set out the conditions in which abortion is lawful in Victoria, in similar terms to the later decision in the Wald case in NSW.

       In practice surgical abortion is available to women in cities and some larger towns in Victoria but less accessible to rural women. Medical abortion using **methotrexate/misoprostol** is available from a small number of individual practitioners and clinics. **Mifepristone** is not currently available in Victoria.

Virginia – rated F by **NARAL**. Virginia outlaws abortions as early as 12 weeks. This ban has been deemed unconstitutional because it makes no provision for a woman's health. No abortion may be performed after the second trimester unless three physicians certify in writing that continuing the pregnancy is likely to result in the woman's death or severe impairment of her health. It also requires that life support measures be available in case the fetus is viable. No abortion may be performed until at least 24 hours after the physician or licensed professional under his direct supervision tells the woman, either in person or by telephone, the nature, risks, and alternatives to the procedure intended, the gestational age of the fetus and offers her state-prepared materials to read. No state funds used for family planning may be used to counsel or refer women for abortion. State family planning services extend until two years after the delivery of a baby. The insurance plan for state employees may not cover abortion unless the woman's life is endangered, the pregnancy is the result of a reported rape or incest or a physician certifies that the fetus has a severe defect. Only physicians are allowed to perform legal abortions and they are subject to regulations and restrictions not placed on other physicians performing other procedures. Any person or medical facility may refuse in writing to participate in abortion care based on personal, ethical, moral or religious grounds. Hospitals may refuse on religious grounds to provide contraceptive information. Public funding for abortion is limited to those cases in which the woman's life or health is endangered, the pregnancy is the result of rape or incest or the fetus has a severe abnormality. A minor woman under 18 must obtain the notarized signed written consent from one parent or other authorized person with whom she lives and who has responsibility for her at least 24 hours prior to having an abortion. This may be waived in cases of rape, incest or medical emergency. In each of these instances, it must be reported. A waiver may also be obtained by judicial order.

Vulva – the external female genitalia.

W

Wendy

I was 20 and had just finished teachers' college when I met Harald. It wasn't long before we were an item. At first we used condoms and then I decided to start taking the pill. I guess I was less experienced than most girls my age, I'd had sex with only one other person before Harald and I was embarrassed about going to the doctor for a prescription. A friend gave me a pack of pills and told me how to take them, while I summoned up enough courage to make an appointment at the student health clinic. What she didn't tell me was not to rely on the pill for the first two weeks. When my period didn't come at the end of the pack it took a while for the penny to drop – I was pregnant.

We talked about it and Harald said he wanted me to have the baby and we should get married. I knew that although I hadn't wanted to be pregnant that I didn't like the idea of abortion and I definitely couldn't go through a pregnancy and give a baby up for adoption. I wasn't very sure about getting married either, I was wanting to be a teacher and travel before I had a family, but I didn't see any other options. We did it very quietly and didn't tell our families until afterwards. That's when my mother dropped the bombshell. I knew I had a brother who had died when he was two years old, before I was born, and now she told me he had severe hemophilia. There was a 50% chance that I was a hemophilia carrier and that if the baby was a boy he would be haemophiliac like my brother, because that's the way this disease is inherited.

By this time I was more than three months pregnant. Harold and I talked and talked and in the end decided we would just go ahead with the pregnancy and accept what God gave us. After a lot of worry that turned out to be a wonderful baby girl whom we named Britt. She is four now; she and I have both been tested and we are both carriers for hemophilia.

This experience brought me and Harald closer together and we have a good marriage. I am planning to start my own teaching career when Britt starts school next year. When she was two we considered another pregnancy and we discussed hemophilia with a counselor. We were told that we could have a test at 12 weeks of pregnancy and if I was found to be having a son with hemophilia I could have an abortion. Both Harald and I knew we could never do that and so instead of trying for another baby I had a sterilization operation. We are both thankful for the one beautiful child we have.

W

Wainer, Bertram and Jo – Prominent Australian abortion activists in the 1960s and 70s. Dr Bertram Wainer challenged the assumption in Victoria that abortion in any circumstances was illegal and uncovered extensive police corruption in the provision of illegal abortions in the state. His campaigning led to the prosecution of Dr Davidson and the Menhennitt ruling in Victoria. The Wainers established the Fertility Control Clinic in Melbourne in 1972.

Wald case – Legal case brought in 1971 in NSW, Australia, against Dr Wald who was charged with performing an illegal abortion. Justice Levine determined that abortions in NSW are lawful where 'the operation was necessary to preserve the woman involved from serious danger to her life or physical or mental health which the continuance of the pregnancy would entail' and the treating doctor may take in to account 'the effects of economic or social stress that may be pertaining to the time.'

Wall – a structure that encloses, divides or protects a body part, eg uterine wall.

Warfarin – a drug used to treat and prevent abnormal blood clotting. When used in the first trimester of pregnancy, it can cause birth defects or abortion.

Washington – rated A+ by **NARAL**. Washington has affirmed the right to reproductive choice in the state code. No abortion may be performed after viability unless it is necessary to preserve the woman's life or health. Only physicians are allowed to perform legal abortions in Washington. No individual or private medical facility may be compelled to participate in abortion services. Washington allows public funds to be used for abortion. Washington law also protects against clinic obstruction or violence .Any insurance plan offering prescription drug coverage in Washington must also offer the same coverage for contraceptives. Pharmacists are allowed to dispense emergency contraception to women without a prescription. Sexual assault victims have access to emergency contraception in hospital emergency rooms.

Webster vs. Reproductive Health Services – Finding of the Court was that a state can require doctors to test for viability and reiterated that public buildings and public funds may not be used for abortion except when the mother's life is endangered.

West Virginia – rated B by **NARAL**. West Virginia has not repealed its pre-Roe ban on abortion but the West Virginia Constitution offers greater protection for the right to choose than does the US Constitution. A woman may not obtain an abortion until at least 24 hours after her healthcare provider informs her orally of the gestational age of the fetus, the description and risks of the intended procedure and the risks of carrying the pregnancy to term. In addition, at least 24 hours prior to abortion, the woman must receive a state-mandated lecture of state-prepared materials. Healthcare personnel and facilities may refuse to participate in sterilization procedures or in other actions contrary to their religious or moral beliefs as long as they promptly inform the patient and cooperate in transferring care. State employees who object on religious grounds may refuse to participate in offering family planning services. If a health insurance plan in West Virginia covers prescription drugs, it must also cover all FDA approved contraception and out-patient services for contraception. Public funds can be used for abortion if it is considered medically necessary or the pregnancy is the result of rape or incest.

Western Australia – In Western Australia in 1998, following an attempted prosecution of two doctors and a major public campaign, a new section 199 was inserted in to the Criminal Code (WA). In combination with amendments to the Health Act 1911 and the Criminal Code of 1913, Western Australia now has a fairly comprehensive statutory system dealing with the performance of abortions, including late abortions. These sections would appear to apply equally to both surgical and medical abortion. The law requires that abortions be performed by a registered medical practitioner, in circumstances where the woman will suffer 'serious personal, family or social consequences' or 'serious danger' exists to the physical or mental health of the woman. The woman must give 'informed consent' and must be provided with specified advice, information and referral to a free-standing clinic.

WHO – see World Health Organization

Wisconsin – rated F by **NARAL**. Wisconsin has not repealed its pre-Roe ban on abortion. No abortion may be performed after viability unless it is necessary to preserve the life or health of the woman. In such case, the method most likely to preserve the life of the fetus must be chosen unless it further endangers the woman. An abortion may not be performed until at least 24 hours after a physician tells the woman, in person, the gestational age and description of the fetus, the details of the abortion procedure and its risks, the medical risks of her pregnancy, the availability of technology for viewing her fetus or hearing the heartbeat, and that if the fetus is viable, the physician must do all necessary to try to preserve its life. She is also required to receive a state-mandated lecture of state-prepared materials, again at least 24 hours prior to the abortion. No public funds may be used to counsel or refer for abortion unless the woman's life is in danger. Only physicians may perform legal abortions and they are subject to regulations and restrictions that do not apply to other physicians doing other procedures. Any doctor or hospital employee may refuse on moral or religious grounds to participate in abortion services; the refusal must be in writing. No hospital or other facility may be required to participate in abortion; this must be written. Similarly, physicians, hospitals and hospital employees may refuse to participate in sterilization procedures. This must also be written. No state employee, who objects because of personal beliefs, may be required to participate in offering family planning services. Insurance plans in Wisconsin may not include coverage for abortion; such coverage may only be obtained by a separate rider from those companies offering it at an additional premium cost. Public funding of abortion is restricted to those instances where the abortion is necessary to preserve the life or health of the woman or the pregnancy is the result of reported rape or incest. A minor woman under 18 may not obtain an abortion without the written informed consent of one parent or adult family member. This provision may be waived if the pregnancy is the result of rape or incest, in medical emergencies and by judicial order. Wisconsin affords legal protection against clinic obstruction or violence. Wisconsin law requires that employers providing insurance coverage for prescription drugs also provide equitable coverage for contraception.

Withdrawal – coitus interruptus, or removing the penis from the vagina just prior to ejaculation. Marginally effective as a method of contraception.

Womb – popular term for uterus.

Women's Ephemera Collection – collection of newsletters, flyers, reports and news clippings about the grassroots women's liberation movement. It is housed in the Northwestern University Library's C. D. McCormick Library of Special Collections.

Women's Liberation – beginning in 1967 and 1968, groups of women joined together, primarily in American cities, identified issues such as sexuality, relationships between men and women, and housework as collective issues and thereby political. These groups used lobbying and militant tactics to make demands known. Originally primarily made up of white women, they were later joined by women of color. Black women's liberation groups also arose within the African American protest organizations.

World Health Organization – has expressed strong support for safe, legal and accessible abortion to be available for all women. In 2003 re-iterated this in its publication of *Technical and Policy Guidelines for Safe Abortion*. In 2005 included **mifepristone** and **misoprostol** on its list of essential medications for developing countries.

Wyoming – rated D by **NARAL.** Wyoming bans post-viability abortion unless the woman's life or health are in imminent danger. Only physicians are allowed to perform legal abortions. Any person may refuse to participate in abortion services and no private hospital or facility can be required to participate in abortion. The institutions are required to notify a patient of their policy. Wyoming prohibits the use of public funds for abortion unless the abortion is necessary to preserve the life of the woman or the pregnancy is the result of reported rape or incest. A minor woman may not have an abortion until at least 48 hours after the physician obtains written consent from one parent. The only waiver of this provision is through a judicial order.

X

My story is not pretty; that is why I don't want you to know my name. I was fifteen and a half when I found I was pregnant. My cousin is the father; we'd been messing around since we were about twelve and we didn't think you could get pregnant with a relative. We'd have big family gatherings and Corey and I'd sneak off to the hayloft or a far pasture. Oh yeah, we'd ride the horses and stuff, too, but mostly we wanted to mess around.

I was so scared when I did the home pregnancy test with my girlfriend. She bought it and all. I knew my folks would kill me when they found out. My girlfriend was great – she went to the doctor and asked lots of questions for me. Her Mom thought she went for her allergies, so we kept it secret. The doctor told her there is a clinic in Fargo that does abortions, but that's way the other side of the state and I couldn't get there, even if I could get the money.

So, I did what I had to. . . I told my folks, but I said that it was a cowboy that I met at the rodeo we went to a couple months before. Like I thought, they hit the ceiling. Daddy whipped me with his belt until Momma yelled at him to stop because he'd hurt the baby. They sent me to my room and I just crawled under the bed and waited until they decided what they were going to do with me. I didn't have to wait long; two hours later, they called me down and told me I'd have to get the next morning. "I won't have no whores in my house," my Daddy yelled.

I cried all night and I was so scared. In fact, I've been scared most of the time ever since. Next day, I called my girlfriend and she came and got me. She didn't dare tell her parents what it was about, so she just said my Daddy was whaling on me and I needed a place to sleep for a couple days. It was my girlfriend suggested we talk to Mrs. Brown – you know, she brought me to you. Mrs. Brown was our English teacher and she always let us know we could bring our problems to her. I bet nobody else ever brought her such a whopper though.

Mrs. Brown has been great. It's like she's the only one who really cares about me. She made some phone calls and I stayed at my friend's house for a couple days, while Mrs. Brown found someplace for me to go. She had friends in Bismarck who said they'd take me and Mrs. Brown drove me there, herself. Her friends are good people and we made a deal: I'd help with their two little boys until my baby came and they'd take care of me and the baby until about a month after the baby was born. Then we'd talk about what to do next. They arranged that I went to court to get an order that said my parents weren't taking care of me anymore and then I was able to get Medicaid to cover me and the baby.

They did what they said and they were kind. I like their kids and it wasn't hard helping with them. I actually stayed until my Theo (I read a book of names and it said Theodora meant a gift of God) was six months, then they said they thought few I should find a better job. Well, it's easy to say find a better job, but if you are not quite seventeen and you have a baby, you can only get the jobs regular folks won't take. The only good thing was that a church ran a daycare that would take little babies, or we'd have been plumb out of luck. I ended up working two jobs regular and babysitting on my days off. I met another single mom and we traded off babysitting when the daycare was closed. Theo and I lived in a room we rented from two other women.

Today, Theo is six and just about to start school and I keep thinking that will make it better. It can't be any harder unless one of us was sick.

If I could have, I'd have had an abortion and today, even though I love Theo with all my heart and I'd die before I'd let anyone hurt her, I still think it would have been best if I could have had the abortion. Then I could have finished high school and my first baby wouldn't have gone hungry sometimes and I'd have been able to have pretty little dresses for her and just generally we'd be better taken care of. Good people are all that has kept Theo and me from dying in a horse stall, and I mean it.

X

X chromosome –one of the sex chromosomes. Females have two X chromosomes, males have one X and one Y
Xeromenia – the usual symptoms of menstruation without menstrual blood flow.
X-linked – determined by a gene located on the X chromosome

Y

Yvonne

When I was young, I thought nothing bad could ever happen to me and so I lived in a very reckless way. I did drugs, drank too much and slept around. Of course, so did a lot of other people. With all of that, I thought that birth control would harm my body by whacking out all my hormones, so I refused to use it. Sure, I'd use rubbers sometimes, but lots of times, we'd just think it wouldn't happen.

It did happen, though and by the time I was twenty-five, I'd had six abortions. They were all early suck outs and I thought it was kind of like having your teeth cleaned. In my late twenties, I sort of went straight. I mean, I got a regular job, stopped doing drugs, except for a rare joint, and only had a few drinks on a weekend night with a date. I got choosier about sleeping with a guy, too. I had seen an old girl hanging out in the bar and I sure didn't want to end up like her.

I met Todd when I was twenty-nine and I couldn't believe that any guy could treat me so good. He was the real works – educated, good job and he even owned his own house. I couldn't believe he'd even look at me. We started dating and with his encouragement, I went back to school. Just a few classes to see how I'd do. I loved it and within a year, Todd and I got married and I was going to college, fulltime. Everything was rosy until we started trying to have a family. I kept having miscarriages. After the third, the doctor said that it was not common, but maybe it was related to all the abortions I had. I was crushed.

We started the paperwork to apply for an adopted baby and last year, we finally got word that our baby was waiting for us. His name is Ethan and we love him to bits. Now, here I am, pregnant again. We'll keep our fingers crossed

Y

Y chromosome – male sex chromosome
Yolk – the nutrient portion of the egg.
Yuzpe method of emergency contraception – see contraceptives, emergency

Z

Zoe

You'd think given how much talk there is about sex in the media, and how it's now perfectly okay to be a single mother, that people would be more laid back about talking about abortion. But they aren't are they? Last year when there was so much discussion about RU 486, I was at a dinner party. Six men, six women, not all of us partnered. The talk turned to the politics of the abortion pill and I said brightly, well, I've taken it – twice! I found it much less traumatic than a surgical abortion. Despite a considerable amount of alcohol on board, everyone else shifted uncomfortably and not one other woman supported me although later one told me that she had had an abortion and admired me talking about it. She said she was a practicing Catholic and that's why she couldn't speak up. So abortion even though it's legal is still one of those things 'we don't talk about' as my dear mother would have said.

I had my first abortion when I was 20. I was a student, I was living at home and I could not afford the pill from my allowance. I got pregnant at a party, after far too much to drink, with someone I hardly knew, in the marital bed of the party giver's parents, who obviously were away for the weekend. Not a very original story, I admit, but one it seems many of our politicians, though they did the same things themselves as students, think is scandalous. There was no way I could have had a baby, no way in fact that I even thought of it as a baby. I was able to borrow the money, not a lot but a lot for me then, from the brother of a friend – in exchange for sex with him. And me a doctor's daughter! I had a suction abortion done at nine weeks and the clinic fitted me for a diaphragm as well.

I graduated and went to London and lo, at 25, became pregnant again, in a short but intense relationship with an older man who of course was not interested in either marriage or children. Neither was I, frankly, at that point. By then medical abortion was available, I was able to have the RU 486 in a clinic and have what seemed like the first day of a heavy period with really supportive clinic staff around me. They were very keen on contraception, rightly so, and gave me a year's supply of the pill for free. So they were not to blame when I forgot to take it with me on a weekend away about six months later and became pregnant again.

Reading over this, I feel I sound callous and foolish. But I know that most of my friends were the same. I did have sex – often, I liked having sex, and if you have sex you can become pregnant. No contraception is 100% and in more short term relationships it can be hard to bring up the subject before it's too late. In the area I worked in, magazine production, short term relationships were normal, as were one night stands.

The third abortion was in the same clinic I'd been to before. I saw the same doctor, a woman, and she spent a lot of time talking to me. She persuaded me to have the hormone rod put in my arm – a new device then – and I have it still. Since then I've come back home. I am not in a steady relationship at present. I'm 38, with a good job and only a small mortgage on a house I love in an inner city suburb. I'm not sure that even if I found a perfect partner I'd want a child with him, and I'm aware that time is running out.

This doesn't worry me – I have a job I enjoy, a hectic social life and a niece who is gorgeous but demanding. In a way I regret having had three abortions but I see it as a personal price I had to pay to be in control of my own life.

Z

Zidovudine – antiretroviral drug used in treatment of HIV/AIDS. Also known as AZT.
Zygote – single fertilized cell formed by the union of a sperm and an egg.

Conclusion

In the previous A – Z listings, you will have found the answers to many questions about abortion, including much of the history, short biographies of the people who have been prominent advocates on both sides of the abortion issue, laws passed that relate to abortion and reproductive rights, the legality and availability of both abortion and contraception by states, and accurate, up-to-date medical information about medical and surgical abortion techniques, contraceptive options, and the advantages and side-effects of both. This information is accurate and verifiable and is evidence-based.

In the appendices, we have provided resources to help you find an abortion clinic or adoption help near you, if your own doctor cannot help you with this. We have also listed a number of good books that you might want to read to find out more about a particular aspect of this issue.

No one is pro-abortion, just as it is a misnomer to call a person who advocates the death penalty but opposes abortion, pro-life. The ultimate answer to the problem is to try to reduce the number of unwanted pregnancies. This can be done with reasonable success by making sure that women have access to and knowledge about effective and reliable contraception. In a secular democracy that advocates freedom of speech and religion, definition of the moment at which life commences is rightly left either to scientific proof (current estimate of conscious neural activity puts this at somewhere between 26 and 29 weeks gestation) or the philosophic and/or religious tradition of the individual involved. The morality of one group should be not legislated as the dominant morality of all, when there is no consensus about the specifics involved. Just as we have freedom of speech, surely women should be guaranteed the right of ownership of their own bodies and the governance thereof. Men enjoy this right without question.

We firmly believe that a woman has the right to control her own reproduction and that without this right, not only will there be the personal tragedies of unwanted pregnancies, but also the problems of children reared in poverty and the increased maternal and infant morbidity and mortality that accompanies a lack of access to reproductive choice and technology.

The text of this book presents facts, accurate and verifiable, and is not our opinion. It is fair, though, that we express our personal views here in this concluding paragraph. We trained in Ireland, at a time when contraception was illegal there. Even so, we convened classes in the non-Catholic maternity hospital to learn about contraception and medically necessary abortion because it was accepted that these were important to women's health and that we, who would be practicing in many areas of the world, should not be unschooled in this important area of medicine. This attitude of tolerance for the beliefs of others has ever since informed our medical practices and our individual approaches to life.

References

Books

Craig, Barbara H. and O'Brien, David M. Abortion and American Politics. Chatham Publishing, Chatham, NJ 1993

Faux, Marian. Crusaders: Voices from the Abortion Front. Birch Lane Press, New York, 1990

Feldman, David M. Birth Control in Jewish Law: Marital Relations, Contraception and Abortion as set forth in the classic texts of Jewish Law. New York University Press. New York. 1968

Gorney, Cynthia. Articles of Faith: the frontline history of the abortion wars. Simon and Schuster, New York. 1998.

Hull, NEH and Hoffer, Peter C. Roe v. Wade: the Abortion Rights Controversy in American History. University Press of Kansas, Lawrence. 2001

Hull, NEH, Hoffer, Williamjames, and Hoffer, Peter C.: The Abortion Rights Controversy in America: A Legal Reader. University of North Carolina Press, Chapel Hill. 2004

Mohr, James C. Abortion in America: the Origins and Evolution of National Policy. Oxford University Press, New York. 1978

Noonan, John T, Jr Editor. The Morality of Abortion: Legal and Historical Perspectives. Harvard University Press, Cambridge. 1970.

Reagan, Leslie J. When Abortion Was a Crime: Women, Medicine and the Law in the United States, 1867-1973. University of California Press, Berkeley and Los Angeles, 1997.

Rowland, Debran. The Boundaries of Her Body: the Troubling History of Women's Rights in America. Sphinx Publishing, Napierville. 2004.

Solinger, Ricky, editor. Abortion Wars: a half century of struggle, 1950-2000. University of California Press, Berkeley and Los Angeles. 1998.

Articles

Bankole, Akinrinola, Singh, Susheela, and Haas, Taylor. Characteristics of Women Who Obtain Induced Abortion: a Worldwide Review. International Family Planning Perspectives. 1999 25(2):68-77

Editorial Staff, Emergency Contraception: prudes and prejudice. The Lancet. July2, 2005. Vol 366.

Jones, Rachel K, Darroch, Jacqueline E and Henshaw, Stanley. Patterns in the Socioeconomic Characteristics of Women Obtaining Abortions in 2000-2001. Perspectives on Sexual and Reproductive Health. 2002, 34(5):226

Lee, Susan J, JD; Ralston, Henry J P; Drey, Eleanor, A; Partridge, John C; and Rosen, Mark. Fetal Pain: a Systematic Multidisciplinary Review of the Evidence. JAMA. Aug. 2005, 294(8):947-954.

Kulier R et al Medical methods for First Trimester Abortion. The Cochrane Database of Systematic Reviewsa 2006 Issue 2.

National Vital Statistics Report, Feb. 12, 2002, 50(5)

O'Dwyer, Erin. Aussies Fly Overseas to Get Banned Abortion Pill. Sydney. Sun Herald. April 12, 2005, page 9

Specific Web articles

Abortion Data: Trends, Crime, Welfare, Risk. www.religioustolerance.org

About Abortion Procedures. www.fwhc.org/abortion/ab-procedures.htm

Abortion Law Development.
www.policyalmanac.org/culture/archive/crs_abortion_overview.shtml

Contraception Report. www.naral.org

Federal Legislation, www.naral.org/legislation

Trupin, Suzanne R, MD, Moreno, Carey. Medical Abortion: Overview and Management. Medscape General Medicine. 2002, 4(1) www.medscape.com

Violence by anti-abortion activists. www.holysmoke.org/fem/fem0542.htm

Jewish Attitudes towards Abortion.
http://caae.phil.cmu.edu/Cavalier/Forum/abortion/background/judaism1.html
http://www.israelnews.com

Islam and Abortion. www.crescentlife.com/family%20matters/islam_and_abortion.htm

Abortion in Canada. www.theglobeandmail.com/series/morgentaler

www.commondreams.org/views01/1108-06.htm

www.cbc.ca/news/background/abortion

Web references

www.canadian-health-network.ca
www.womenshealthmatters.ca/centres/sex/abortion/index.html
www.lifesite.net
www.physiciansforlife.ca
www.pregnancycenters.org
www.ncln.ca
www.birthright.org
www.lifecanada.org
www.menandabortion.com
www.prochoiceactionnetwork-canada.org/canada.html
www.caral.ca/layout/index.html
www.cbctrust.com
www.morgentaler.ca
www.NARAL.org
www.plannedparenthood.org
www.nnaf.org
www.morgentaler.ca
www.pathfinder.org
www.bpas.org
www.mariestopes.org.uk
www.childrenbychoice.org.au
www.plannedparenthood.com.au

www.fpa.net.au
www.shinesa.org.au
www.mariestopes.com.au
www.guttmacher.org

Resources

UNITED STATES AND CANADA

Planned Parenthood – www.plannedparenthood.org or phone 1-800-230-PLAN (1-800-230-7526)

For those seeking abortions services:
www.naral.org or phone 202-973-3000 primarily USA and Canada

Community Abortion Information and Resources – information about clinics and funding for abortion in the USA – phone 1-888-644-2247

National Abortion Federation – www.nnaf.org information about clinics in the USA or Canada phone 800-772-9100 in the USA or 800-424-2280 in Canada

Morgentaler Clinics – www.morgentaler.ca eight abortion clinics in Canada

Canadian Abortion Rights Action League – www.caral.ca phone hotline 888-642-2725 provides a directory of clinics in Canada as well as information on the laws in each province.

Crisis Pregnancy Resources – i.e. offering counseling and/or services relating to carrying the pregnancy and keeping the baby or arranging adoption:

Bethany Christian Services – operates a large adoption agency – www.bethany.org or phone 1-800-238-4269

Birthright – www.birthright.com gives resources in the USA, Canada, South Africa and Columbia. 888-205-3132

Care Net – www.carenet.org 800-395-HELP (800-395-4357)

Harbor House – www.harborhouse.org referral through Care Net 800-395-HELP

Heartbeat International – www.heartbeatinternational.org international listings of resources. 800-395-HELP

America's Crisis Pregnancy Helpline – www.thehelpline.org 800-672-2296

Resources

AUSTRALIA

NATIONAL

Abortion Information and Access
www.abortion.org.au

QLD

Children by Choice
07 3357 5570
www.childrenbychoice.org.au
info@childrenbychoice.org.au

Family Planning Queensland
07 3250 0240
www.fpq.com.au

NSW

Family Planning NSW
FPA Healthline 1300 658 886
www.fpahealth.org.au

VIC

Family Planning Victoria
03 9257 0100
www.fpv.org.au

Women's Health Victoria
www.whv.org.au
03 9662 3755

TAS

Family Planning Tasmania
03 6228 5244
http://www.fpt.asn.au/
Hobart Women's Health Centre
03 6231 3212
www.hwhc.com.au

ACT

Sexual Health and Family Planning ACT
02 6247 3077
http://www.shfpact.org.au/

Women's Centre for Health Matters
02 6290 2166
www.wchm.org.au

SA

Pregnancy Advisory Centre
08 8347 4955
www.pregnancyadvisorycentre.com.au

SHINE
(Sexual Health Information, Networking and Education)
08 8431 5177
http://www.shinesa.org.au/

WA

ALRA WA
http://users.bigpond.net.au/alra/index.htm
wa.alra@bigpond.net.au

Family Planning Western Australia
08 9227 6177
http://www.fpwa.org.au/

NT

Family Planning Welfare NT
08 8948 0144
http://www.fpwnt.com.au/

Printed in the United States
134514LV00001B/32/A